Probing The Mind
And Other Guiding Symptoms

(A Blueprint for Success)

Probing The Mind And Other Guiding Symptoms

(A Blueprint for Success)

S.M. Gunvante

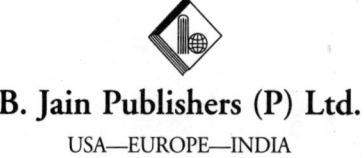

B. Jain Publishers (P) Ltd.
USA—EUROPE—INDIA

PROBING THE MIND AND OTHER GUIDING SYMPTOMS

First Edition: 1990
Second Revised & Enlarged Edition: April, 1992
9th Impression: 2015

All rights reserved. No part of this book may be reproduced, stored in a retrieval system or transmitted, in any form or by any means, mechanical, photocopying, recording or otherwise, without any prior written permission of the publisher.

© with the Publishers

Published by Kuldeep Jain for
B. JAIN PUBLISHERS (P) LTD.
1921/10, Chuna Mandi, Paharganj, New Delhi 110 055 (INDIA)
Tel.: +91-11-4567 1000   Fax: +91-11-4567 1010
Email: info@bjain.com   Website: **www.bjain.com**

Printed in India by
B.B Press, Noida

ISBN: 978-81-319-0837-2

WITH GRATEFUL THANKS TO

Dr. Vishpala Parthasarathy for the encouragement and guidance given to me in writing this booklet; and to

Dr. Rajan Sankaran for instilling immense confidence in classical Homoeopathy, and in the prime importance of Mentals in understanding the image of the patient (through Video cases, talks and discussions), and to R. & K.T. Thakur Charitable Trust for giving me the opportunity to serve in the O.P.D. of the Trust's AFAC Homoeopathic Centre, St. Antony's Road, Chembur, Bombay. The copyright in this book vests with them.

—*S.M. Gunavante*

CONTENTS

		Page
	Preface	1
1	Probing the Mind of Patients	3
2	Guiding Symptoms	9
3	Evaluation or Hierarcy of symptoms	15
4	Repertorisation	19
5	Minimum Syndrome of the Maximum Value	23
	Genius of Remedies Nux Vomica	26
6	A Blueprint for Success	29
7	Personality-Group-wise Rubrics of Mind	31
8	Unlocking the Patient's Mind	37
9	Rubrics corresponding to the complaints described in Section 8.	57
10	Repertory Page-wise Rubrics giving Serial No. of complaints against which they appear in Section 8.	63
11	Do not neglect Objective Symptoms	69
	Appendix: Trend of thought necessary....J.T. Kent	76
	References	77
	Recommended Essential Reading	77

PREFACE

Homoeopathy has achieved many marvellous cures guided by the *Law of Similars*. What are the symptoms which should guide the prescriber in the application of this Law has been specified by Hahnemann in a number of Aphorisms of the Organon. In Aph. 210 he has said that "in all cases of disease we are called on to cure, the state of the patient's disposition is to be particularly noted, along with the totality of symptoms." In Aph. 211 he emphasises that "the state of the disposition of the patient often chiefly determines the selection of the homoeopathic remedy."

The absolute correctness of Hahnemann's directions is being witnessed by us daily in every case where the "change in the state of mind and disposition" (Aph. 213) has been taken into account in arriving at the remedy. It is not possible in this short preface to cite such examples.

As every homoeopathic physician knows, eliciting the characteristic "physical" symptoms is comparatively easy, and at any rate, it is not as difficult as understanding the state of mind and disposition. The result is that physicians who make an earnest attempt to understand the mental state of the patient are very few. This is due to the simple reason that they have not cared to train themselves in this art, probably excusing themselves that it is time-consuming. Consequently, patients are deprived of the best benefit which Homoeopathy as a science is capable of giving.

Something had to be done to remedy this situation. The author therefore, contributed an article (in two parts) to the *Indian Journal of Homoeopathic Medicine*, Bombay, under the title *"Probing the Mind of Patients"*. Since this article was appreciated by a number of students, the Editor of the Journal advised me to bring out the ideas in a booklet. I, however, felt that the booklet will be incomplete unless clear advice on how to elicit other Guiding Symptoms is also given; hence this aspect has been covered.

The main object of this booklet is to lay down a track by following which the physician's task in understanding the state of mind and disposition of the patient (or changes therein) is made very easy. The steps to be taken for this purpose are described in Section I herein under the title "Probing the Mind."

A few illustrative cases are also given to show how the method can be put into practice.

In view of the fact that many students complain of getting confused when "taking the case", we felt the necessity of outlining how to elicit the other symptoms which complete the "totality of the case" such as the *physical generals, causations, concomitants* and the *peculiar*, uncommon and characteristic symptoms (sometimes called Key-notes). This feature will be found in Section 2. (In Section 7 Personality-wise Groupings of Rubrics as discussed in Section 1 are given).

Evaluation or Hierarchy of symptoms for purposes of repertorisation or finding the remedy—a task of crucial importance in our search for the similimum—is discussed in Section 3. The technique of Repertorisation "without tears" is explained in Section 4. In Section 5 we stress the immense usefulness of knowing the "Minimum Syndrome of the Maximum Value" of the remedies. In Section 6 we present a Blueprint for Success including a few hints on dosage and management of the case.

When this book was being given to B. Jain publishers for publication it was felt that its usefulness could be enhanced if we added two more Sections, viz. "Unlocking the Patient's Mind" and " Do not neglect Objective Symptoms." The former Section shows how patients narrate their complaints (in thier own words) and how each situation can be interpreted into a corresponding Rubric in the Repertory. It is our experience that the more a physician thinks of complaints or situations of patients in terms Rubrics, the more easily and quickly he can arrive at the simillimum. Over 200 of such examples have been given, and the reader is required to think for himself as to the Rubric each situation represents; and the answers are given in the second part of this Section. Section 9 gives a list of Objective signs and symptoms which are of no mean importance in helping the physician to find the simillimum.

We hope that Practitioners will find this revised and enlarged edition to be of much practical value. Suggestions for improvement will be gratefully received.

Moraya Villa,   —*S. M. Gunavante*
12th Road, Khar,
Bombay, 400 052.
10th June, 1992.

1
Probing the Mind of Patients

If we go through Kent's Repertory, and even more so, the Synthetic Repertory, our head reels at the enormous number and variety of rubrics in the chapter on Mind. One gets confused as to where to begin and where to end while taking the case. In the opinion of the writer, the only way to bring this enormous knowledge within the working capacity of the average physician is to broadly classify the rubrics into certain well-defined Groups which can be easily remembered. On referring to these Groups as pivotal points, the various related rubrics (which are facets of the related Groups-Personality) come before us at a glance. There Personality-Groups with their rubrics are given in the Section 7 of this booklet. To enable the reader to fix the Personality-Groups in his mind, the ruling characteristics of each of these Groups are given below.

Ruling Characteristics of Personality Groups

Natural Disposition
I Domineering (Go-getter)
II Mild (Sensitive)
III Anxious, fearful, timid
IV Restlessness
V Planning and thinking
VI Lascivious
VII Unsocial behaviour (qualities society does not approve)
VIII Unsocial traits
IX Destructiveness

Altered Disposition
X Sad, melancholy
XI Extreme effects (expressions of extreme intensity like Shock, Anguish, Rage)
XII Dullness (Weak mind)
XIII Imbecile (Idiocy)
XIV Alienation, mental
XV Delusions; strong, fixed feelings
XVI Habits, Obsessions.
XVII Causations; Ailments from
XVIII Agg. or Amel. from

How to use the Group Classifications: In Aph.104 of the Oraganon Hahnemann states: "When the picture of the disease, whatever be its kind, is once accurately sketched, the most difficult part of the task is accomplished..." How to do this is described by him in Aph. 84: " The patient details the history of his sufferings...how he has behaved... and (the physician observes) the altered or unusual character about him... Keeping silence himself, the physician allows the patient to say all that he has to say, and refrains from interrupting him." These instructions are unexceptionable and no one has found it possible or necessary to improve upon them. The best plan for us in taking the case, therefore, is to ask the patient to narrate his entire life situation, including his mental, emotional disposition, hopes, aspirations and frustrations, and their effects on him. He should be asked to cite actual instances of his behaviour to enable us to judge his reactions in their proper context. He should be advised to tell even such peculiar sensations and "feelings" (delusions) which he might consider laughable and unimportant. He should be told that these strange and peculiar symptoms are in fact most important for us in selecting the curative remedy. Thus, having been briefed adequately for narrating his case, the patient give us a fairly good picture of his personality and his present emotional make-up. All this helps us to make a *tentative* decision about the "Personality Group" or Groups (out of those given above) to which he belongs.

It is the physician's turn now to interrogate the patient for more details required to get a complete *image* of the patient which, as Kent says, is the soul of Hahnemenn's teaching. Quite often even after proper briefing the patients are not able to give full details about themselves. It is at this stage that many failures in eliciting "full details" occur, because the doctor gets confused as to what questions to ask. He meanders from one line of enquiry (according to a set pattern formed by habit) to another. Such questioning becomes purposeless, a wild goose chase, and ineffective. As a result, his conclusions about the patient's state of mind become erroneous.

This situation can be avoided if the physician refers to the rubrics in one or the other of the Personality Groups depending upon the nature of the emotional or mental disposition to which the patient predominantly belongs, as revealed when the patient was telling his story. Suppose you have categorised the patient as belonging predominantly to Group I (domineering), you should now question him to ascertain as to which one or more of the several rubrics given under this Group conform with his mental disposition. Of course, the questions should be tactfully worded in order to elicit his response. For example, instead of asking whether he is domineering, ask him how he deals with subordinates who are inefficient and on the other side, with superious who are exacting. An effective method is to pose hypothetical situations in day-to-day life (relevant to each rubric in that Group) and ask how he would react to them—by open anger, vexation felt internally, by reserved displeasure (suppressed anger), by brooding, by dwelling on the event for long, by losing temper with family or subordinates, by weeping in the privacy of his room, by anorexia, taciturnity or by sleeplessness, and so on. As far as possible, an attempt should be made to elicit actual instances of the type of behaviour under discussion for, confirmation.

While eliciting his response to various rubrics under the Group concerned, the patient may reveal that rubrics under some other Groups also apply to him. All these rubrics (under the predominant Group or otherwise) which apply to the patient in different degree or intensity, should be noted (with marks of intensity) in the right hand margin of the Case Record. It is important to note that *cases cannot come exclusively under one Group.* Therefore, while we start with questions based on Rubrics in the predominant Group, if symptoms belonging to another Group are found to be strong, they too should be noted. In, fact, it is advisable to elicit his response to a few plausible rubrics under other Groups as well. This procedure gives us an assurance that we are on the right track, and permits us to correct it if we are mistaken.

This type of questioning on a right track eliminates the chance of our missing some important aspects (components) of the case, and makes our case as broad-based and complete as possible. Of course, the procedure is not mechanical. A lot of Judgement on the part of the physician is called for in determining the relative value of the symptoms (expressed through rubrics) while taking them for repertorisation. It is an essential requirement while using the rubrics for repertorisation that one *should not neglect to search for sub-rubric which may be appropriate* to the case. The Synthetic Repertory abounds in such Sub-rubrics which are also accompanied by valuable cross-references.

In general, in probing the mind, we should not neglect to elicit the *patient's state of mind* in regard to the deepest instincts of life and survival, such as desire for company, approval and appreciation, sensitivity to hurt, accomplishment or frustration, sexual impulse and gratification, the manner in which he seeks relief and relaxation from the strains and stresses of life (e.g., music, religion, indifference, etc.). The physician should develop an appropriate repertoire of questions through which the patient's mind can be peeped into.

The author feels certain that with the faithful application of this procedure, the case-taking becomes more efficient (especially the mental symptoms), less time-consuming and satisfactory to all concerned. The procedure may appear cumbersome to begin with, but after the first 15 or 20 cases it will be found to be easy, smooth, less tedious and, what is more, to yield magnificent dividends in the form of accurate prescriptions.

We shall illustrate the application of this method through a few cases.

Case 1:- The mother complained that her 7 years old son had violent anger. Whenever he wanted anything he demanded it, and was very impatient till he got it. He was very obstinate. If mother did not comply immediately, he would weep and say "You do not love me; you better kill me." He was worse in a warm room, and had a craving for sweets. He had bed-wetting.

Discussion: As the mother was narrating her complaint, it was obvious that the boy came under Personality Group I (domineering). On referring to the rubrics under this Group, we were able to ask questions and get confirmation from the mother about a number of rubrics, viz. Anger violent (39), Impatient (600), Haughty (572), Obstinate (788), Dictatorial (398). The boy's "Weeping in children" came under Group XI. Further confirmation of Lyco (which emerged after repertorisation) came from "Warm agg". and "Desires sweets". The chief complaint of Bed-wetting was also covered by Lyco.

Case 2: Padmakshi, age 14, complained that though intelligent she could not concentrate on her studies, was very slow in everything and forgot what she had studied the previous day. Was irritable if awakened early for school. Was sleepy during menses which were apt to be profuse. Had no self confidence and was averse to mental exertion. Being the only daughter, she was afraid of being alone if the parents returned late from their jobs.

Discussion: It was obvious that her mental state came under Personality Groups XII, "Dullness of mind". On referring to the rubrics under this Group we were able to "direct" the questioning on a track and elicit information on a number of other aspects of her mental state (apart from inability to Concentrate), viz. Concentration difficult, learns with difficulty (158), Memory weak for what she has read (739), Work, averse to mental(1096), Slow (936), Confidence, want of (159)-All these rubrics are under Group IX. "Fear of being alone" only is under Group III. Phosphorus was the remedy and it helped her.

Case 3: Cheated by his business partner, Mr. A. G. had to withdraw from his Partnership firm at the age of 55. After this event he became morose, brooding over the past events all the while, full of remorse for trusting his partner too much. He became sleepless after the first sleep, and once the sleep was broken, he would not fall asleep for 2 to 3 hours. He lost hope of ever getting out of this insomnia and began to say that death would be welcome instead. He would not talk much with anyone, and yet would liven up from his profound sadness when in company.

Discussion: This patient came under Personality Group X for profound depression. The rubrics in this Groups guided us to direct the questioning and obtain some more relevant information about his mental state, which we could straightway convert into Rubrics, viz. Brooding (115), Despair (391), Remorse (830), Loathing of life (710), Sad when alone (871), Talk, indisposed to (986). A.F. Mortification (21) is under Group XVII. AURUM which emerged covers sleeplessness after waking.

It should be pointed out that Case Taking is best done when the physician exercises his power of observation to the maximum. This involves great insight into human nature, an ability to judge the manner in which and the extent to which the patient's fears, thoughts, demeanour, reactions depart form the normal. These impressions are gleaned not so much by questioning as by engaging him in natural conversation about his work, family life, hopes, disappointments and frustrations, etc. This ability is not easily acquired, but the constant use of the Rubrics under each Personality Group will go a long way to help develop this ability. After all, to use Stuart Close's expression, a prescription can be made only on those symptoms which have their counterpart or similar in the Materia Medica, and the Repertory. The Personality Groups will make one thoroughly familiar with many Rubrics which otherwise would be seen or referred to only by chance.

2
Guiding Symptoms

Hahnemann declared in Aph. 18 that the "sum of all the symptoms and conditions in each individual case of disease must by the *sole indication*, the sole guide to direct us in the choice of a remedy." In Aph.7 he says that the totality of symptoms must be the principal, indeed the only thing the physician has to take note of in every case of disease. Masters like Stuart Close, Roberts and Kent have thrown much light on what this "totality" means. We give here the salient points from their teachings.

Totality does not mean numerical sum of all the symptoms; all symptoms are not of equal value. Symptoms of disease do not help us to individualise the patient or his remedy. The individualising symptoms are always "the more striking, singular, uncommon and peculiar (characteristic) signs and symptoms, and they should chiefly and almost solely be kept in view." (Aph. 153). A. Pulford says: these strange and peculiar symptoms contain the core of the drug; they are constant in ALL provers of that drug. They never vary, no matter who or what the individual is. The remaining numerous symptoms of a drug vary with each individual and in the same individual at different times. So, they cannot help us to arrive at the similimum. (The striking, strange and peculiar symptoms almost approximate to our idea of the "Minimum Syndrome of the Maximum Value," about which we shall give examples in Section 5 of this booklet). We shall give a brief list of such individualising symptoms, so that the reader does not overlook to check them up while taking the case.

Symptoms are classified broadly into 10 types, viz. (1) Mental Generals, (2) Physical Generals. (A General symptom is one which applies to the patient as a whole, and not to this parts alone). (3) Particulars - applicable to parts of body only. (4) Peculiar, uncommon and characteristic symptoms (sometimes called Keynotes). (5) Causation of complaint. (6) Concomitants. (7) Common symptoms. (8) Objective symptoms. (9) Pathological symptoms. (10) "Accidental symptoms" all these are described below in a little more detail.

(1) **Mental symptoms** - have been considered in Section 1 already.

(2) **Physical Generals:** They fall into several parts. No case-taking is complete unless an effort is made to elicit as many of them as possible. They are:

(a) **Thermal modality:** Better or worse from Heat or Cold (as applied to the whole person (general). from Sun, hot or cold bathing; draft of air.
(b) **Time modality:** *General* and *Particular*: Exact time of recurrence of complaint; morning, forenoon; mid-day or mid-night; afternoon, evening, before mid-night; after mid-night, etc. Also whether Agg. during Full Moon or New Moon.
(c) **Periodicity of complaint:** Alternate days, weekly, yearly, etc.
(d) **Modalities of Circumstances,** such as Agg. or Amel. (General or Particular)—Whether the complaint, or the patient as a whole is better or worse before, or during, or After each of the following circumstances:
(i) Eating (ii) Drinking (iii) Stool (iv) Urination (v) Coition (vi) Lying on back, on left side, or right; or on abdomen; (vii) Sleep (viii) Menses (ix) Exertion, physical or mental (x) Hanging down of limbs or raising them (xi) Looking up or down or side-ways (xii) Touch, even slight (xiii) Pressure simple, or hard (xiv) Lying with head high or low (xv) Nature of sleep, or loss of sleep (xvi) Loss of vital fluids-blood, semen, leucorrhoea (xvii) Stooping, or standing straight (xviii) Overlifting (xix) Rubbing (xx) Motion, slow or fast or at perfect rest (motionless) (xxi) Strong odours (xxii) Darkness (xxiii) Thunderstorms: (xxiv) Noise, sensitive to (xxv) Whether discharges agg. or amel.
(e) **Appetite and thirst:** Whether normal, extreme or wanting. When and under what circumstances.
(f) **Craving for and Aversion** to (*or aggravation from*): Items of food or drink: Study various items of food and drink listed in Synthetic Repertory (Vol.II).
(g) **Nature of sleep:** Disturbed, sleepiness, sleeplessness before or after midnight; sleeplessness after waking; sleepless from activity of mind (brooding, planning); sleep unrefreshing in the morning, etc. Also position in sleep.
(h) **Dreams** which are more or less repeated, or vivid, frightful, pleasant, etc.
(i) **Sexual impulse:** *Desire strong or weak* and complaints of sexual function.
(j) **Menstrual disorders**—Leucorrhoea, etc.
(k) **Perspiration:** Whether profuse, or partial (or only on particular parts of the body, e.g., scalp); or if it stains or stiffens the linen.
(l) **Trembling:** As a concomitant of emotional or physical complaints.

(3) **Particular Symptoms:** Particulars are symptoms which relate only to parts of the body. They are least in importance because they are not complete—the provings could not be pushed to the point of producing all possible Particulars. Yet they are important, provided they are "qualified" by aggravation or amelioration or they appear as Concomitants. They have been either ill-used (neglected)—because Kent gave last place to them, after Mentals and Phy. Generals - or abused (wrongly used). Kent's advice to "Go from Generals to Particulars" only means that you take Particulars *last*. He said, he was "devoting his life to the growth and infilling and perfecting of this work", showing forth "all the particulars with the circumstances connected with them." If Particulars were unimportant Kent would not have laboured to collect them in such large numbers as we find in his Repertory. He has attached only two conditions to their use: they should be qualified by a modality and, secondly they should not stand contrary to the mentals and physical generals. Used in this way they guide us quickly to the similimum. Experience has amply confirmed this fact.

(4) **Peculiar, Uncommon, Characteristic Symptoms:** When symptoms pertaining to the disease and pathology are separated from the total anemnesis of the case, what is left is symptoms of the patient. These will be common if not qualified by a modality or concomitant. Those which are qualified can be regarded as peculiar, individualising symptoms. Guernsey termed them as "Keynotes". According to Guernsey the Keynote is simply the predominating symptom or feature which directs attention to the *totalilty*. He did not teach prescribing on a single symptom. Kent advised that if the Keynote, which is often a characteristic, is taken as *final*, and the generals do not conform, then will come the *failures*. A few peculiar, indiviualising symptoms are given.

(a) **Side of the body:** right, left or diagonal; or from Right to left or left to right; or alternating sides.

(b) **Direction or extension of the symptoms:** Downward, outward, upward, radiating. In other words, the part from which the pains extend and the parts to which they do so (given at the end of the main rubrics in Kent's Repert). The "Directions" will be found in Boger-Boenninghausen's Rep. (p. 892).

(c) **Alternating states:** Diarrhoea alternating with constipation; Eczema with Asthma; physical with mental, etc.

(d) **Onset and Exit of symptoms (K.1377):** Whether increasing gradually and decreasing slowly; increasing suddenly and decreasing suddenly, etc.

(e) **Area of pain:** Whether in a spot (K.1385), or radiating in all directions; or whether they are not in a fixed place and are wandering from one area to another (1389).

(f) **Discharges:** (Sweat, Expectoration, Urine, Coryza, Leucorrhoea, Stool): Their consistency, colour, odour, acrid or bland.

(g) **Taste:** Alterations in, sweet, sour, saltish, insipid, taste of the expectoration.

(h) **Discolouration:** Of face, lips, around the mouth, circumscribed, etc., bluish, greenish, pale, cyanotic, red - under various conditions like during headache, chill, menses, cough, excitement, toothache.

(i) **Hanging down or raising of limb:** Agg. or amel. of pains from (K.1009)

(j) **Nausea:** At the thought, sight or smell of food.

(5) **Causation:** Aetiology is one of the most important aspects of case-taking, and no complaint should be passed over without probing deeply for the cause - mental, physical or the history of illness, or strong Family History of Asthma, Tuberculosis, Cancer, Diabetis, Heart Disease.

• (6) **Concomitants:** Disease is a disturbance of the vital force which pervades the whole organism. This disturbance manifests itself as disorders in various parts of the body at the same time. They are not separate diseases, but a group of symptoms. The chief complaint represents the most suffering, while the auxiliary, associated or concomitant symptoms are also part of the *toality*. It is often found that the concomitant symptoms are not only co-existent, but they seemingly have no relation to the leading symptoms from the standpoint of theoretical pathology. We might almost term them as unreasonable attendants of the case in hand. H.A. Roberts says: "The concomitant symptom is to the totality what the condition of aggravation or amelioration is to the single symptom. It is the differentiating factor". Concomitants, when identified, are very useful in limiting our search for the similimum to a few remedies, *e.g.*, headache with coryza (K. 138), vomiting on coughing (532), involuntary urination, convulsion during (K. 659).

(7) **Common Symptoms:** Common symptoms are such as are pathognomonic of diseases and or pathology. As such they are common to many remedies and are found in large rubrics in our repertories, e.g., constipation, nausea, irritability, memory weak, weeping, fever, burning pains, paralytic pains, weakness. Kent devoted his life to bring them down as sub—rubrics with their respective modalities as we find

Guiding Symptoms

in his Repertory, *i.e.*, such as were confirmed clinically. We still find a number of remedies in these large "general" rubrics of common symptoms which are not yet qualified. These remedies cannot be ignored on that account, as they are useful all the same even when we do not find them in the "qualified' sub-rubrics. We could use the modalities in the Generalities Chapter to qualify such "common" remedies. Hahnemann has acknowledged that he owes these to the genius of Boenninghausen. They are useful when we have to find remedies pertaining to certain conditions, (distension, hiccough), or certain locations (forehead, knee), or organs (spleen, heart, lung) or sides of body (right, left) or sensations (heaviness, jerking, stitching). One should not neglect to use them whenever necessary. For this purpose Boger—Boenninghausen Repertory is also very useful.

(8) **Objective Symptoms:** I cannot do better than quote from Boger's Synoptic key: "Next in order comes the entire objective aspect or expression of the sickness. This should especially include the—Facial expression, Demeanour, Nervous excitability, Sensibility, Restlessness or Torpor, State of the secretions and any abnormal colouring or odour that may be present. This includes flapping of alae nasi, wrinkled forehead, tongue coated or fissured or mapped, face flushed or pale, one cheek (or foot) hot and the other cold. Blood when it is fluid and fails to clot is a peculiar, as it reflects a change in the whole economy which makes it a general. A list of objective symptoms is given in Section 9.

(9) **Pathological Symptoms:** There are a number of pathological rubrics in the Repertory. Obviously, they are drawn from clinical experience and cannot be exhaustive. What is more, if we make them the basis, we prescribe for results, for endings, and not for things first, not for the cause. They cannot help us to individualise the remedy.

(10) **Accidental Symptoms:** Stuart Close says: "The true Totality" is more than the mere numerical totality or whole number of the symptoms. It may even exclude some of the particular symptoms if they cannot, at the time, be logically related to the case. Such symptoms are called "accidental symptoms" and are not allowed to influence the choice of the remedy. Totality is that concrete form which the symptoms take when they stand forth as an individuality recognisable by anyone who is familiar with the drugs".

He says again: "Totality is more than the mere aggregate of its constituent symptoms... As the parts of a machine cannot be thrown together in any haphazard manner, but each must be fitted to each other part in a certain definite relation according to a preconceived plan or design—"assembled" as the mechanics say—so the symptoms of a case must be "assembled" in such a manner that they constitute a recognisable identity, as we recognise the personality of a friend.

3
Evaluation or Hierarchy of Symptoms

A case could be taken in detail, but unless it is followed by a proper evaluation of symptoms an important step towards the similimum will be missed. This step is as crucial as it is confusing and many failures can be attributed to this difficulty. The issue has become complicated because even the masters have given advices which differ from one another. In the opinion of this writer it would become easy for practitioners if they understand the two aspects of evaluation, both of which are equally sound; one is the *ideal evaluation*, and the second is *practical evaluation*.

Ideal Evaluation: Following Hahnemann's emphasis that the 'state of disposition of the patient often chiefly determines the selection... as being decidedly characteristic symptom which can least of all remain concealed from the accurately observing physician" (Aph.211), Kent gave the highest ranking to the *mental symptoms*, next the *physical generals*, then the *peculiar* and *characteristics*, ending with *particulars*. Boger on the other hand, following Boenninghausen's approach gave the highest ranking to *modalities*, then *mentals*, followed by *sensations*, next the *objective aspect* and lastly the *parts affected* (Synoptic Key). At the same time Boger points out that the *actual differentiating factor may belong to any rubric whatsoever*.

Practical Evaluation: The physician should always aim at and never desist from making every effort at using the ideal evaluation in his practice in every case, because it has been found to give deep and long lasting cures even of difficult cases. The practical evaluation we are suggesting here is only intended to guide the neophyte in making a *start* at a lower level than the ideal, instead of losing his way, losing confidence and taking to Allopathy. We should realise that the average physician labours under two limitations, firstly his own lack of ability in taking the case fully and, secondly, "the inability of the patient to express symptoms in the language that would best indicate the real nature of his case" as Kent said.

In these circumstances, our advice to the neophyte is as follows. Firstly, Margaret Tyler, Gibson Miller, Yingling and others have stressed that a symptom to be considered as a pointer to the remedy must be of *equal grade* in both the patient and the remedy. This means that while taking the case we must note those symptoms which are *intensely* felt by the patient, and therefore, *spontaneously* expressed, and those which are also clear and *unambiguous*, by underlining them or with marks 2 or 3. This procedure will help us to concentrate only on a few symptoms which are high ranking, instead of wasting our time on all and sundry symptoms which cannot help us to find the simillimum.

Secondly, as Boger has said, "the differentiating factor may belong to any rubric whatsoever." This means that our choice of the symptoms for repertorisation should not be restricted to the "theoretical or ideal" evaluation, if it is not possible in a case and should be extended to any group of symptoms provided: (i) they characterise the patient, not the disease - they are outstanding Generals and Peculiars, or (ii) they are well marked Particulars with the three aspects strongly marked, viz. location, sensation and a strong modality (with a Causation and/or Concomitant if possible). For example, lumbar pain agg. from stooping and worse during menses in a hot patient was speedily cured with Sulphur 10 M one dose. Remember Kent's assertion: "A strong General will overrule any number of weak Particulars; also, "a number of strong Particulars must not be neglected on account of one or even more weak Generals."

In short, the neophyte should carefully note which of the symptoms (Mentals, Physical generals, qualified Particulars, Modalities, Sensations, Causations and Concomitants) are *outstanding, intense* and *clear* in the patient, and do his repertorisation with them. This applies to all cases where the *present* symptoms are available.

In chronic cases it sometimes happens that the patient comes up with some acute complaint. Gibson Miller and Boger have said: "Ranking close behind, or even at times taking precedence of the peculiar and general symptoms, must be placed the *last-appearing* symptoms of a case. These symptoms to be of any real importance, must of course be outstanding and definite, and if so, they are always of the first importance in the choice of the remedy ... such a remedy will modify the symptoms and open up the way for other remedies."

On the other hand, Dunham, Kent and Miller have pointed to cases where the *old symptoms* have been suppressed and the whole character of disease has changed. In these circumstances it becomes necessary at times to give the original symptoms the higher rank and to be guided by them to the exclusion of those now present. Dunham's well-known case of deafness cured by Mezereum is an example. Gibson Miller cites two more such cases, one his own and the other of Kent.

Some points need to be stressed before concluding this Section.
(i) As clearly pointed out by all Masters (and experienced even today in many cases), the changes in mental disposition or the mental state are so

very important in arriving at the similimum, that if correctly understood and applied, they alone can lead to the correct remedy. To neglect to do our best to understand the patient's mind would thus amount to missing a vital part of the "Totality"—like seeing "Hamlet" without the Prince. Of course, we should make sure that they are clear and outstanding.

(ii) It is possible that one can go wrong in understanding the mind of a patient. Therefore, it is advisable to obtain confirmation of the remedy arrived at on the basis of the mind, from the Physical Generals such as thermal and other modalities, cravings and aversions, sleep or dreams, etc.

(iii) A remedy which stands on the solid foundation of Mentals and Physical Generals is definitely the simillimum; and one can confidently expect favourable results.

(iv) On the other hand, a remedy based on Physical Generals alone, or supported by Qualified Particulars, can only be the next best, (but never as good as the one based on Mentals and Physical Generals) and you cannot be sure what the result will be.

(v) H.A. Roberts neatly sums up the answer to the problem of therapeutical selection of the remedy. He says: Hahnemann never slighted any symptoms of a case in making a prescription... It is inconceivable that he ever did keynote prescribing... nor did his thorough mind eliminate the chief complaints in building up the symptom image. Our way, too, must lie in the golden mean between these two points... If we can find a remedy that has the "more striking, particular, unusual and peculiar (characteristic) signs and symptoms of the case" and in addition covers the chief complaint as well, we may consider ourselves as having a sound basis for the prescription of the simillimum.

(vi) The chief complaint is generally a Partricular (relating to a part of the body). Hence, H.A. Robert's advice follows the line advocated by Boger in his Synoptic key. This is in flat contradiction to the advice of Kent to give primary importance to Mentals, the Physical Generals and Particulars following. Experiences of many Homoeopaths (as well as various Aphorisms in Organon) confirm the correctness of Kent's advice. (See Kent's observations at page 76). Therefore, until he masters the art of forming the image of the patient through his mental disposition, the average physician would have to follow the "Practical Evaluation" suggested above. It is needless to emphasise, however, that one should not be surprised at failure if a prescription ignores the Generals.

(vii) Particulars with strong modalities, or peculiar sensations such as "splinter" pains, or specific "direction" or "extension" of pains, or peculiar

Concomitants, should not be neglected when they are clear and outstanding in the patient.

(viii) In cases where pathology is advanced and characteristic symptoms are wanting or unclear, the possibility of lesser known (ill proved) remedies proving useful should be thoroughly explored.

(ix) Not all cases call for the same approach. The artistic physician decides which of these approaches will suit an individual case. This art (intuition) is a result of deep study, sufficient experience and reflection on the results obtained in each case to draw appropriate conclusions.

4
Repertorisation

In a cry of exasperation Kent said (How to Study the Repertory): "If Boenninghausen used a Repertory with the limited remedies then proved, how much more do we need to consult it!" Unfortunately, many practitioners do not know *how to use* the Repertory *easily* and *quickly* in spite of Margaret Tyler's wonderful booklet on this subject.

The secret of getting quick and accurate results from repertorisation is: (i) Arrange the outstanding and characteristic symptoms according to their rank (General, Peculiar and *well marked*); (ii) Take the first two top-ranking symptoms/rubrics as "Eliminative" rubrics; (iii) Write out the 2 and 3 mark remedies which are *common, i.e.* which are in both these two top-ranking rubrics, with their marks in a Tabular form, as shown below; (iv) Work out the marks for the remaining rubrics, only in respect of the remedies emerging in the preceding step—ignoring (eliminating) *all* other remedies which are not common to the first two rubrics; (v) Find out which remedy (out of the several) covers all the rubrics and which remedy gets the highest total marks. (vi) If there is a tie, study the remedies in the Materia Medica, or elicit additional symptoms which will help you to differentiate between the remedies.

Care should be taken to see that the first two eliminative rubrics are indispensable to the case but not too short; otherwise, you may throw out the real simillimum by a careless choice of the eliminative rubrics.

Here is an example of repertorisation of a case of Mucous Colitis. Note that the first two rubrics are taken as "Eliminative Rubrics", and only those remedies which are common to them have been considered for the remaining rubrics.

Rubrics	Page KR.	Arg.n.	Ars.	Lyc.	Med.
A.F. Anticipation (Very anxious when boss calls for an urgent report)	4	2	1	1	1
Great craving for sweets	486	3	1	3	2
Anxiety, time is set, if a	8	2	-	-	1
Agg. warn	1412	2	-	2	-
Dreams of snakes	1243	2	-	-	-
Abdomen, pain cramping before stool	576	3	2	-	-
Stool, bloody	635	2	3	2	2
Stool, mucous	639	<u>3</u>	2	-	-

19/8

Guy Buckley Stearns advises: "In using the repertory, *symptoms as unrelated as possible* should be selected (as eliminative). Only a few should be used... the few remedies that come out in the repertorial analysis should be compared in the Materia medica.

Tyler's advice is worthy of note; "You will find, as you work down, that one drug stands out more and more prominently - it may not be in all the rubrics, but it has *got to be in all the important ones, i.e.,* those best marked in the patient and of highest grade.

A point on which many neophytes get confused, when selecting the similimum, is what to do when some leading symptoms of a remedy are not present in a patient, though that remedy appears to be the similimum in many other respects. The answer lies in the fact that in every case our aim is to fit the patient's symptoms into the remedy (*i.e.,* those symptoms which are *positively* found in him). It is *wrong to fit the remedy into the patient.* It is just not possible, nor necessary, that the large number of symptoms of a remedy - even those most leading in it - can be found in a particular patient. A Lachesis patient need not necessarily be "suspicious" or "religious", and a Sepia patient need not be "indifferent". However, certain Keynotes of a remedy are indispensable, (such as Worse from heat of Lachesis, Worse from motion of Bryonia, Mild and yielding nature of Pulsatilla), which all students of Materia medica know about.

Finally, it must be realised that the best curative work can come only when the *image* of the patient (his peculiar mental and physical state) matches with the *Genius* of the remedy. This necessitates our knowing and *understanding* the materia medica, on which Kent laid much stress. If we understand the core, the essence, the soul of remedies, we will not be baffled when we are confronted with a maze of symptoms, some of which may not be in tune with the outstanding characteristics of any one remedy. The key to understanding remedies lies in Kent's advice: "Get the strange, strong peculiar symptoms, and then SEE TO IT THAT THERE ARE NO GENERALS IN THE CASE THAT OPPOSE OR CONTRADICT. Also, do not expect a remedy that has the generals must have all the little symptoms... Learn to omit the useless, common particulars". We shall discuss how to understand the genius of remedies, in the next section.

Repertorisation—Advanced method:

Dr. H.C. Allen in his Preface to "Keynotes and Characteristics" says that the practitioner must have a knowledge of the peculiar, uncommon or sufficiently characteristic symptoms of the remedies, which may be used as as a *pivotal point of comparison.* This laconic advice is pregnant with

Repertorisation

meaning which gives us wonderful results. For example, a child was brought with albumen in urine, oedematous face, etc., which the Allopathic doctors called the "Nephrotic syndrome". The peculiar symptoms for the Homeopathic prescription were: the mother had terrible fear in the seventh month of pregnancy as a number of goondas came threatening to kill her husband in a business dispute. Then the child has fear of darkness, and fear of being alone. He would scream if the mother was not with him (she being in the kitchen) whenever he woke up from sleep in the morning or in the afternoon. He is now 3 years old and sleeps on the abdomen. Whenever a stranger comes to the house, the boy would not leave the lap of the mother or father. The rubrics in this case are: A.F. Fright, Fear of darkness, Fear of strangers. Clings to father or mother. Fear of being alone. (Just a month before the present trouble started, the child had fallen in a tank, and was rescued just in time. He is still afraid of water). The most peculiar symptom in this case may be taken as "Fear of being alone". If we use this rubric as the PIVOTAL POINT OF COMPARISON with the next rubric, "Fear of darkness", we find Stramonium emerging strongly. Then we check up if Stram is present in the other rubrics, one by one and we see that Stram covers the case fully. If we recognise that Fear is the dominant feature of this case, this knowledge will help us to discard most of the remedies in "Fear of being alone" at a glance. But this method can be used only after a lot of repertorisation work, with a good knowledge of the peculiar characteristics of remedies, plus finger - tip knowledge of the differentiating features, such as thermal state, cravings and aversions, outstanding mentals, and other symptoms given in section 2 of this book.

5
Minimum Syndrome of Maximum Value

Hahnemann has told us in Aph. 118 of the Organon that "every medicine exhibits Peculiar actions on the human frame, which are not produced in exactly the same manner by any other medicinal substance..... of a different kind." Again, in Aph. 119 he says:" Each of these substances produces alterations in the health of human beings in a peculiar, different, yet determinate manner, so as to preclude the possibility of confounding one with the other." This is so far as the power inherent in medicines is concerned. As regards the question of matching those powers with a patient, Aph. 210 says: "...in all cases of disease we are called on to cure, the state of the patient's disposition is to be particularly noted, along with the totality of the symptoms..." H.A. Roberts has thrown clear light on what constitutes "Totality." He says, "...no disease can be represented by a *single symptom*. The character of the drug is represented not by a single effect, but by a *group of effects*. Further, "No medicine can cure any disease unless it acts upon all the diseased parts, whether directly or indirectly..... One organ cannot suffer alone any more than one cell can suffer by itself." Therefore, very often the *concomitant circumstance* is of great importance to the whole case than the expressed sensation..."

What is the nature of symptoms which should guide us to the curative remedy, apart from the "state of disposition"? Hahnemann clarifies in Aph. 153: "The more striking, singular, uncommon and peculiar (characteristic) signs and symptoms...are chiefly and almost solely to be kept in view."

From the above discussion we now draw the following conclusions:
1) Each remedy has *peculiar characteristics* which preclude the posibility of confounding it with another.
2) The character of each drug is represented by a *group of effects*.
3) In understanding the genius of a remedy—based on the peculiar characteristics in the *Group of effects* (totality)—we have to take into consideration (i) the mental disposition and the (ii) peculiar, uncommon characteristics which naturally relate to the physical sphere. They will necessarily be "Physical Generals" since the Particulars are born out of the constitutional predisposition of the prover/patient and disappear or are palliated only when the constitutional state improves (Pulford).

4) Since the symptoms of mental disposition and the peculiar Physical Generals of a particular remedy cannot be very many, we term this group as the "Minimum Syndrome".

Kent has said: It is sometimes possible to abbreviate the anemnesis by selecting one symptom, the key to the case, but this should be seldom attempted. It is often convenient to take a group of three or four essentials. Hering had found that three important characteristics, clearly defined, pointing to one remedy, seldom failed...and he had tested this in hundreds of cases. Sir John Wier, Dr. Paschero and Dr. Candegabe have found that the "Minimum Syndrome of Maximum Value", (a typical group or combination of symptoms) represent the vital essence of a drug. The *"Minimum Syndrome"* may there-fore comprise a group of symptoms—mental, physical general, peculiar uncommon and qualified particular—all singular and outstanding.

5) Next in selecting one remedy in preference to another, a number of masters like Margaret Tyler, Elizabeth Hubbard, Dr. E.J.Lee and Yingling have emphatically stated that the *most prominent symptoms of the patient* must not only be in the remedy but they *should be one of the most prominent of the remedy*. In understanding remedies, therefore, we should concentrate on those chracteristics which are most prominent, i.e. of *"Maximum Value."* A remedy could be said to be of maximum value against a rubric (symptom) if it is the only remedy or one of the very few high ranking remedies against that rubric. There are quite a few single remedy rubrics, or rubrics with very few high ranking remedies in Kent's or Synthetic Repertory. Such rubrics if found equally strong in a patient, could straightaway single out that remedy as a possible similimum (provided other symptoms agree). (Symptoms classified in this manner, under each Remedy, are given in "synthetic Mat. Medica of Mind from MacRepertory" by Dr. Hari Singh (Indian Book & Periodicals Syndicate, P.O. Box 2525, New Delhi, 110 005).

6) The formula for drawing up the "Minimum Sydrome of the Maximum Value" of any remedy would thus be: A *small (Minimum) group* of marked Mental and Physical Generals, as well as Peculiar Uncommon symptoms, which at the same time are of *outstanding importance (Maximum Value.)* Such a group of symptoms of a remedy will have very few competing remedies of the same value. When even a few of the symptoms in this group are taken together there can be little possibility of confounding this Group identity with another remedy.

Minimum Syndrome

A few examples of such "Minimum Syndrome..." which we would like to call the Genius of Remedies will be in order:

(a) "And now, to sum up. If you get a patient with severe stitching pains, worse for the slightest movement, worse for sitting up; better for pressure; very thirsty for long drinks of cold water; very irritable; angry and not only angry, but with sufferings increased by being disturbed mentally or physically; white tongue; in delirium "wants to go home" (even when at home); busy in his dreams and in delirium with his everyday business—with these you can administer BRYONIA and-bet on the result! (Margaret Tyler in "Drug Pictures")

(b) Dr. Kirpal Singh Bakshi says: "I have cured cases of chronic Epistaxis, Sciatica, Rheumatic Arthritis and Malignant Hypertension with CINA when symptoms of ravenous hunger and clean tongue were present." A somewhat enlarged group of CINA would be: Children, irritable, nervous and peevish, who resent being touched or even looked at; obstinate, permit no one to approach them; Pale face usually associated with dark rings about eyes. Grinds teeth during sleep. Pale face even during hot stage. Spasmodic...whooping cough with tonic convulsions. Bores finger into nose. Asthenopia from defective accommodation.

(c) On seeing the hyperactive child in my consulting room I felt like I was sitting at the centre of a tremendous hurricane. Nothing that the parent told me could give me a clearer picture than the one I saw for myself. Once I learned further that she loved music and would dance for hours, that she craved salty and spicy food, and was averse to meat, there was no question in my mind that TARENTULA HISP, was the indicated remedy... and it produced a profound improvement.

-Dr.S.Kipnis, U.S.A.

(d) A man who has undergone or is going through much stress; has been very industrious, under the burden of unusual responsibility, becomes intolerant of contradiction or with a sense of justice becomes taciturn; sense of duty not done brings on pangs of remorse with anxiety of conscience. He must offer pooja and prayers: enjoys immense relief from his cares from soft, classical music (bhajans); else develops loathing of life, desires death, has suicidal thoughts. Despairs from the pains. Has a forsaken feeling. Craves milk and is averse to meat. His physical correlations may be hypertrophy of heart (cardio-vascular complaints), or uterus hemiopia, sees only the lower half; enlargement of or pain in the right testes. With some of this Group of symptoms Dr. Rajan Sankaran has cured a number of "incurable" conditions, with AURUM MET, which the writer has seen.

(e) Burning heat, redness, the heat fairly burning the examining fingers, flushed red face and pupils dilated to the limit giving a wild appearance, carotids throbbing violently, pains and sweats coming and going suddenly—these, in a case of renal calculi that had been from pillar to post for four years, was relieved at once and two calculi passed without pain in 24 hours. He went back to hard work and has had no more attacks of renal trouble now for over a year. A single dose of BELL. 10M did the trick. No case like this was ever cured that did not include the small primary pathogenetic group as indicated above. (A.Pulford).

Advantages: The essence, the core or the grand characteristic of *drug pictures* is best and more easily grasped through the "Minimum Syndrome." *"Understanding* the remedy through this method helps us to *Think* of the remedy from the *Synopsis itself,* even while we are taking the case. Thus a knowledge of a few but most characteristic symptoms of a remedy helps us to "direct" our questions purposefully while taking the case. The questioning does not remain "directionless" or "incomplete" (the two pitfalls in case-taking pointed out by Pierre Schmidt). This knowledge also builds up an increasing knowledge of Rubrics in the Repertory with an enhanced ability to compare remedies in the same rubric.

The Genius of "Nux Vomica" is given here as an example. The author is compiling the "Genius" of other Polychrests in the hope that they will be of substantial help to the practitioners.

Genius of Remedies
NUX VOMICA

I   **SYNOPSIS (Identifying Features):**
1. Sedentary life with exhausting mental labour
2. Ambitious, zealous, easily angered and offened, malicious, spiteful, Rage leads to violence.
3. Ardent, fastidious, vehement. Angry from contradiction.
4. Gastric complaints with constipation; ineffectual desire for stool or vomiting or urination.
5. Sleepy in evening; wakes up at 2, 3 or 4 a.m. lies awake for an hour or two, then falls into heavy sleep and awakes late, tired and unrefreshed.

6. Ill effects of disappointments, deceived ambition.
7. Much relieved after stool. With nausea feels, "If only I could vomit I would feel better". The more retching prevails over the vomiting, the more it is Nux.
8. Desire for fats, alcoholic stimulants, pungent things.
9. During labour or rigid, with constant urging to stool and urinate. (Dysmenorrhoea or pain in sacrum also with the same peculiar symptoms)
10. In lumbago must sit up in bed to turn over.
11. Shaking chill, cannot stand the least uncovering, even of part of body. Must be covered well during every stage of fever.
12. Extreme sensitiveness to pain, or trifling ailments, so much, that he "prefers death" to suffering; faints from odours, from every labour pain.

II CAUSATION (A.F.): Mind - Anger, fright, indignation. Deceived ambition. Disappointment, emotional excitement, wounded honour.

III MODALITIES: Aggr. cold, open air (dry), draft, early morning. Coffee, drugs. Purgatives. Liquor, Overeating, Noise; odours; touch; Pressure of clothes at waist; new moon. Suppressed hemorrhoidal flow.

Amel: Evening, while at rest, Damp weather (Caust, Hep, Med) Free discharges, Naps, Hot drinks, Milk, Fats, Moist air, Lying on sides.

IV FOOD & DRINKS: Appetite-thirst:
Emptiness yet aversion to food, Fullness after eating a small quantity.
Craves—Piquant food; beer; fat food, chalk, stimulants,
Amel—Hot drinks (gastralgia)
Disagree—Coffee. tobacco, alcoholic stimulants.

V MIND: Ardent, Zealous, Easy anger, Violent anger, Easily excited, Extremely fastidious, Fault finding, Hurried Impatient, Quarrelsome, Jealous, Malicious, Spiteful, Tenacious, Vehement, Head-strong, Self-willed, Easily offended, Angry when contradicted, Oversensitive to slightest noise, odours, even trifling ailments, Company, averse to, Agg. by mental exertion, Concentration difficult while studying, Suicidal thoughts, but lacks courage, Sudden impulse to kill for a slight offence, Rage leading to deeds of violence, Generosity to strangers, avarice in regard to family.

VI **FEMALE:** Menses profuse, early, protracted, Dysmenorrhoea, Cramps extend to whole body; with constant urging to stool, Inefficient labour pains, with urging to stool or urinate. Menses return at full moon.

MALE: Sexual desire easily excited, cannot be in female company without having emission. Premature ejaculation, Nocturnal emissions.

VII **CHILD:** Snuffles of infants. Frequent and unsuccessful desire for stool, or passes a small quantity at a time. Emaciation with ravenous appetite, Nose stuffed, prevents nursing in infants. Colic from flatulence and constipation. Shreiking at night. Left inguinal hernia in children.

VIII **PECULIAR, UNCOMMON GRAND CHARACTERISTICS:**
1. Hernia—incarcerated or otherwise in children from constipation and crying, especially if they are cross,
2. Colic, renal, right side, extends to genitals,
3. Frequent ineffectual urging to urinate but the urine only dribbles,
4. Heart—Angina pectoris from suppressed piles
5. Abdomen—Swelling of liver from alcoholic excesses, colic, biliary; gall stone colic.
6. Stomach—Nausea while riding in a carriage.
7. Sleep—Sleepiness after eating—cannot use the mind for two or three hour after eating,
8. Drunkenness—Abusive, brutal, striking, jealous, sad, sexual excitement, Desire for suicide.
9. Mind—Shreiking of children at night before epileptic convulsions.
10. Vertigo—at night waking him from sleep; from odour of flowers; with obscuration of vision.
11. Stomach—Vomiting after anger; immediately after drinking; before menses.
12. Bladder—Retention after confinement. Urination involuntary during cough, or laughing, or sneezing.
13. Epilepsy—Aura in stomach, in solar plexus.
14. Kidneys—pain in ureters extends to penis and testes.
15. Hemorrhoidal flow from suppressed; epistaxis, or vomiting bloody, or haemoptysis.
16. Constipation alternating with diarrhoea.

6
A Blueprint for Success

1) Have unshakable faith in the *Law of Similars* as explained in the Organon, "Genius of Homoeopathy" by Stuart Close, "Principles and Art of Cure by Homoeopathy" by H.A.Roberts, "Lectures on Philosophy" by J.T.Kent, "Evaluation of Symptoms" by Gibson Miller.

2) Closely *study articles* by Masters appearing in Journals, as well as cases. Through cases one can learn a lot about the peculiar characteristics of remedies which helped, the different approaches to selecting the remedy, potency and repetition, etc. *Regular contribution* to prominent Homoeopathic journals is a must.

3) Become thoroughly *familiar* with the various *Rubrics* in the Repertory. Use all your spare time for this, so that your work in searching for the similimum becomes easy and quick. A prescription can be made only on those symptoms which have their *counterpart* or *similar* in the Materia Medica (and repertory). Stuart Close.

4) Compile your *own list of leading remedies* and their "Minimum Syndrome of Maximum Value" (Mental, Physical Generals and Peculiars) and have those characteristics at your finger tips. *Update* them every time a case has been cured with any of them.

5) Regular *participation in discussion groups*, at periodical intervals, and at seminars and conventions is worth the time and expense, as you come back with new inspiration and deeper understanding of remedies and philosophical approaches.

6) Follow the procedure outlined herein for (i) *perceiving the image* of the patient, (ii) *analysing* his mental disposition, and (iii) eliciting his Physical Generals, Peculiar symptoms and qualified, outstanding Particulars. (iv) Do not fail to *observe* the peculiar objective symptoms, if any. Mark the intensity of the symptoms with 3,2 and 1 so that it becomes easy for you to be selective.

7) Do the repertorisation work with a Chart (as shown), at least to begin with, and definitely in all complicated cases. Always use the *"eliminative" method*, the first two rubrics being the most important and indispensable to the case.

8) Study and compare the remedies emerging from repertorisation with your knowledge of remedies through the "*Minimum Syndrome of the*

Maximum Value." Check up again with the Materia Medica before arriving at the similimum to be prescribed.

9) *Potency and repetition of dose* is as important as finding the remedy. For this purpose you cannot do better that study Chapter XIII on Homoeopathic Posology in "The Genius of Homoeopathy" by Stuart Close and Chapter XIII on The Dose, in "by Homoeopathy" the Principles and Art of Cure by H.A. Roberts. Also "The Similimum" at p.82 of Kent's "Minor Writings".

10) Kent's twelve *Observations on Management* of the case (and Second Prescription)-Chap.XXXV of Homoeopathic Philosophy-should also be mastered by periodical re-reading. A wrong follow up may spoil all the good work done in selecting the similimum. Study also "The Second Prescription" at p.232 of Kent's "Minor Writings". and "How not to do it " by Maraget Tyler.

11) Chapters XXII to XXX on "*Disease Classification*"—Chronic Miasms —(Principles and Art of Cure by H.A. Roberts) should be *part* of your mental equipment. The ability to identify one or the other of the Chronic Miasms and a knowledge of the remedies needed to treat them is essential for success.

12) Finally, every professional owes a debt to the masters who have left us a rich *heritage*. We have all benefited much from it. This debt can and should be repaid by every one by sharing his own experiences and thoughts with others through articles in journals, and participation in discussion groups and seminars.

**May these twelve Secrets of Success
guide you in your day-to-day work—and
Fortune will surely smile on you.**

7
Personality Groupwise Rubrics on Mind

(From Synthetic Repertory. Those who do not have the Synthetic Repertory may refer to corresponding Rubrics in Kent's Repertory.)

Natural Disposition
GROUP I PERSONALITY (DOMINEERING; GO-GETTER)

0026 Ambition
0026 Amusement, desires
0026 Anger, irascibility
0039 Anger, violent
0101 Audacity
0125 Censorious
0147 Company, desires
0180 Conscientious about trifles
0181 Consolation, kind words agg
0181 Contemptuous
0184 Contradiction, intolerant of
0187 Courageous
0201 Defiant
0398 Dictatorial
0435 Egotism
0446 Excitable
0466 Irritability
0462 Exhilaration
0572 Haughty
0579 Hurry
0593 Ideas, abundant
0600 Impatient
0603 Impetuous
0605 Impolite
0606 Impulsive
0623 Indignation
0630 Industrious
0712 Cannot bear to be looked at (peevish)
0713 Loquacious
0787 Obstinate
0813 Rage, fury
0833 Reserved
0895 Rudeness
0895 Selfish
0981 Sulky
1055 Vanity
1055 Violent, vehement
1059 Vivacious

GROUP II PERSONALITY (MILD, SENSITIVE)

0013 Affectionate
0109 Benevolence
0115 Brooding
0119 Capricious
0127 Cheerful
0181 Consolation amel.
0183 Contented
0189 Credulous
0633 Injustice, cannot support
0677 Jesting
0694 Laughing
0743 Mildness
0761 Moods Changeable
0781 Naive

0791 Offended easily
0810 Quiet disposition
0812 Quiet, wants to be
0835 Rest, desire for
0850 Irresolution
0895 Secretive
0897 Sensitive
0901 Sensitive to noise
0905 Sensitive to odours
0905 Sensitive to pain
0909 Servile

GROUP III PERSONALITY (ANXIOUS, FEARFUL)
0054 Anxiety
0063 Anxiety when alone
0069 Anxiety of conscience
0076 Anxiety with fear
0080 Anxiety about health
0093 Anxiety during sleep
1026 Bashful
0119 Capricious
0121 Cares, worries, full of
0125 Cautious
0142 Clinging to person
0188 Cowardice
0391 Despair
0406 Discouraged
0473 Fearsome
0477 Fear of being alone
0479 Fear of animals
0487 Fear of dark
0487 Fear of death
0493 Fear of impending disease
0511 Fear of misfortune
0962 Fear of Strangers
0546 Forsaken feeling
0549 Frightened easily
0575 Hide, desire to
0578 Horrible things affect him
0761 Moods, Changeable
0764 Morose peevish

0827 Religious
0830 Remorse
0950 Starting, startled
0930 Slowness
0987 Sympathetic
1023 Timidity
1629 Tranquility
1066 Weeping
1096 Witty
1102 Yielding

GROUP IV PERSONALITY (RESTLESSNESS)
0124 Carried, desire to be
0192 Dancing
0446 Excitement, exciteable
0579 Hurry
0600 Impatience
0835 Restlessness
0860 Riding
0861 Rocking
0870 Quick
0928 Singing
1022 Time passes slowly
1030 Travel, desire to
1061 Wander desire to

GROUP V PERSONALITY (PLANNING, THINKING)
0008 Activity
0024 Ambitious
0048 Busy
0141 Clairvoyance
0121 Carefulness
0180 Conscientious
0327 Delusion, has neglected his duty
0492 Exhilaration
0466 Fancies exaltation
0472 Fastidious
0572 Hopeful
0630 Industrious

0792 Optimistic
0792 Overactive
0795 Planning
0800 Precocious
0833 Reserved
0892 Responsibility unusual agg (Phatak's Rep)
0908 Serious, earnest
0997 Theorising
1097 Work, desire for, mental

GROUP VI PERSONALITY (LASCIVIOUS)

0024 Amative
0025 Amorous
0696 Lascivious
0782 Naked, wants to be
0785 Nymphomania
0787 Obscene, Lewd
0892 Satyriasis
0909 Shameless
1013 Thoughts Sexual

GROUP VII PERSONALITY (UNSOCIAL TRAITS)

144 Company, averse to
181 Consolation agg.
413 Disobedience
437 Egotism
440 Hatred
570 Haughty
574 Heedless
674 Jealous
720 Malicious
744 Mischievous
763 Moral feeling, want of
929 Slander, disposition to
949 Squanders
983 Suspicious
1054 Unsympathetic
1055 Vanity

GROUP VIII PERSONALITY (UNSOCIAL BEHAVIOUR)

7 Abusive
102 Avarice
104 Aversion to members of family
107 Bargaining
110 Bite, desire to
119 Capricious
185 Contradictory to speech, intentions are
186 Contrary
190 Cruelty
191 Cursing
200 Deceitful
412 Dishonest
433 Eccentricity
444 Estranged from family
563 Greed
587 Hypocrisy
647 Insolence
687 Kleptomania
706 Liar
806 Quarrelsome
862 Rudeness
895 Selfish
1053 Unfeeling, hard-hearted
1053 Ungrateful
1054 Unreliable

GROUP IX PERSONALITY (DESTRUCTIVE)

0110 Biting, desire
0115 Break things, desire to
0190 Cruelty
0200 Deceitful, sly
0397 Destructive
0402 Discontented
0535 Feigning sick
0682 Kill, desire to
0720 Malicious
0763 Moral feelings, want of
0764 Mischievous

0949 Squanders
0963 Striking
0996 Tears things
1021 Throws things away
1055 Violent

ALTERTED DISPOSITION DURING ILLNESS

GROUP X PERSONALITY (SAD, MELONCHOLY)

0026 Amusement, aversion to
0069 Anxiety of conscience
0104 Averse to family members
0115 Brooding
0117 Averse to business
0144 Company averse to
0181 Consolation agg.
0184 Contradiction, intolerant of
0195 Desire death
0391 Despair
0402 Dissatisfied, Discontented
0431 Dwells on disagreeable occurrences
0546 Forsaken feeling
0576 Homesickness
0607 Inconsolable
0609 Indifferent
0624 Indolence
0688 Lamenting, bemoaning wailing
0710 Loathing of life
0712 Looked at, cannot bear to be
0764 Morose, Cross, fretful
0791 Offended easily
0794 Pessimist
0830 Remorse
0835 Rest, desire for
0864 Sad, depressed
0920 Sighing
0974 Suicidal

0981 Sulky
0986 Taciturn (talk, indisposed to)
1053 Unfortunate feeling
1063 Weary of life
1066 Weeping
1094 Will, loss of

GROUP XI PERSONALITY (UNBEARABLE SHOCKS ANGUISH, RAGE EFFECTS OF)

0039 Anger, violent
0041 Anguish
0566 Grief
0588 Hysteria
0607 Inconsolable
0623 Indignation
0688 Lamenting, bemoaning, wailing
0813 Quieted, cannot be
0813 Rage
0963 Striking
1055 Violent,vehement

GROUP XII PERSONALITY (DULLNESS)

0004 Absorbed (abstraction of mind)
0144 Company averse to
0150 Concentration difficult
0158 Concentration, learning with difficulty
0159 Confidence want of self
0160 Confusion of mind
0416 Dull, comprehension difficult
0537 Foolish behaviour
0539 Forgetful
0595 Ideas, deficiency of
0609 Indifference
0624 Indolence

0733 Memory weak
0745 Mistakes (Writing, speech)
0801 Prostration of mind
0896 Senses dull
0937 Sit, inclination to
0936 Slowness
0966 Stupefaction
0986 Talk, indisposed to
0998 Thinking, averse to
1016 Thoughts, vanishing of
1022 Time, Fritters away
1096 Work, averse to mental
1098 Work, mental, impossible

GROUP XIII PERSONALITY (IMBECILE)
0140 Childish
0398 Development arrested (mental) in children
0413 Disobedience
0537 Foolish
0596 Idiocy
0598 Imbecility
0632 Infantile behaviour

GROUP XIV PERSONALITY (ALIENATION)
0047 Answers incoherent
0201 Delirium
0229 Delusions (all types)
0387 Dementia
0441 Escape, attempts to
0588 Hysteria
0607 Inconsolable
0633 Insanity, madness
0701 Laughing immoderately
0723 Mania
0752 Moaning
0780 Muttering
0892 Schizophrenia
0940 Speech incoherent
0940 Speech nonsensical
0948 Spoken to, averse to being

1032 Unconscious, coma, stupor
1091 Well, says he is, when very sick

GROUP XV PERSONALITY (DELUSIONS-FOR EXAMPLE)
237 Appreciated, she is not
244 Belong to here own family, does not
249 Body, state of his B.
257 Confusion, others will observe her
260 Criticised, she is
335 Persecuted, he is
361 Succeed, he cannot, does everything wrong
372 Unreal, everything seems
377 Voices, hears
387 Wrong, suffered has and many others

GROUP XVI PERSONALITY (HABITS, GESTURES, OBSESSIONS)
SR-I   553 Gestures
SR-I   398 Dipsomania, alcoholism
           776 Morphinism
SR-I   1000 Thoughts, various kinds
SR-I   1026 Touched—different conditions
SR-I   1027 Touch, everything, impelled to (obsession)
           1062 Washing-aversion to, or mania for (obsession)

GROUP XVII PERSONALITY (CAUSATION—AILMENTS FROM)
0013 Anger, vexation
0015 Anticipation
0017 Disappointment
0018 Fright

0019 Grief
0019 Honour, wounded
0020 Disappointment in love
0021 Mortification
0982 (Mental Syts) from suppressed skin disease or haemorrhoids
1031 Trifles, ailments from.. etc., etc.

GROUP XVIII-AGG. OR AMEL

124 Carried, being, amel.
142 Climacteric period agg.
144 Colours, aversion to or charmed by
181 Consolation, kind words, agg.—amel.
186 Conversation agg.
193 Darkness agg.
416 Driving amel. mental symptoms
433 Eating while, amel. of mental symptoms
460 Exercise, mental symptoms amel. by physical exer.
461 Exertion, physical, amel., Mind
461 Exertion, mental, in puberty, agg. mental symptoms
461 Exertion, mental agg.
575 High Places
776 Music agg., amel./ aversion to
790 Occupation amel.
861 Rocking aggr—Amel.
999 Thinking agg. complaints
1021 Thunderstorm, agg. before
1100 Writing agg.
SR-II/ 53 Burns from X-ray (Radio toxaemia)
SR-II 76 Coal Gas
SR-II 242 Fish spoiled
SR-II 253 Meat, bad
SR-II 368 Mushroom poisoning
SR-II 387 Narcotics
SR-II 521 Ptomaine Poisoning
SR-II 601 Smoke inhalation
SR-II 635 Smoking tobacco
636 Tobacco agg
SR-II 639 Tobacco disgust for, to create
SR-II 768 Wounds, dissecting

8
Unlocking The Patient's Mind

In Section I we had said, " The physician should develop an appropriate repertoire of questions through which the patient's mind can be peeped into." We have found that this aspect of interrogation is a great stumbling block to many practitioners, especially those who have newly emerged from the colleges. Therefore, an attempt will be made here to show how one can get over this difficulty of unlocking the mind of patients.

Patients come to us with all kinds of difficulties, sometimes even unbelievable or breathtaking. Many times they do not come out with their full story—for various reasons. Under such circumstances, we cannot be masters of the situation unless we have a thorough knowledge of human sufferings and human psychology and how their counterparts can be identified in the Homoeopathic Materia Medica and the Repertory.

It is well said that "What the mind does not know, the eyes do not see nor the ears can hear." The process of understanding human problems and of comparing them with remedies which match them till we find a fit between the remedy and the patient (says Dr. H.C.Allen in his Therapeutics of Fevers) "shows how difficult it is to take a case unless we have some knowledge of the Materia Medica, and how much an *extensive knowledge of the Materia Medica* aids us in taking the case...(emphasis ours). We however suggest that we substitute the words "Repertory" in place of "Materia Medica". This is because the Materia Medica is so vast that it becomes difficult to compare individual symptoms with those in it, whereas the symptoms of the patient can be reduced to specific rubrics in the Repertory, which can then be studied in their *totality* (synthesis), to come to a few remedies. Reference to the Materia Medica to verify the drug picture and see if it fits the case then becomes easy. This leads us to the conclusion that an *extensive knowledge of the variety of rubrics* in the Repertory helps us more easily to find the matching remedy.

How can we acquire this extensive knowledge? Going through each rubric (several rubrics each day) and pondering over their meaning is one way; but there is a more effective way. That is to see, hear or read of a rubric in action, when it has been used in a case. A rubric once "experienced" in this way cannot be easily forgotten. To experience the rubrics in action we should make it a *habit*, an **invariable practice**, to *observe* and *study* how patients present their complaints, and try again and again to translate or covert their symptoms into appropriate rubrics. Another way of doing the same thing is to study cases reported in journals and try to think out the manner in which the patients must have presented their symptoms, which led the doctor to select certain rubrics. We shall, therefore, narrate what the patients said......, and give in brackets the Rubric corresponding to each situations, with the page number of the Synthetic Repertory, Vol. I

Before proceeding further, let us review briefly *how* we can unlock the patient's mind, permitting the pouring out of his pent-up emotions. The first step is to tell him at the outset, that in order to make a good prescription we need to know him *thoroughly*, including "minor" or "funny" details concerning not merely his physical ailments, but especially his emotional make-up, his anxieties, his fears, disappointments, grief, shock, frustrations, etc. which have profoundly affected him. He should be encouraged to tell everything *voluntarily*, and asked to give actual *instances* of his complaints, His narration of actual events will reveal the *intensity* and **depth** of the *behaviour pattern* and *nature of his responses* to various situations.

When the patient has had his say fully and freely, without interruption, it is our turn to seek *clarification* of those aspects which are *incomplete* or *unclear*. In this situation it becomes necessary to ask *specific questions* which will make him think over the past events in his life which have left *deep impressions* on his mind and emotions.

It is important to remember that symptoms to be considered fit for repertorisation should be outstanding, clear and really morbid, *i.e.*, related to the sick individual, not dependent upon the nature of his disease, not upon his profession or situation in life. For example, it is *natural* for an employee to be yielding to his boss, but if he is given to sudden anger with his boss, it is a *morbid symptom*. Fever in a case of pneumonia cannot rank high among symptoms, but if he is thirstless and resents any disturbance (motion), or lies on the painful side, all these (not related to pneumonia) are *peculiar individualising symptoms*. If a police officer is harsh with suspected criminals, this cannot be a high ranking symptom but if he detests using harsh words or rough treatment with them, his mildness would be out of proportion to the call of his profession. In other words, only those responses which are *out of proportion* or are inappropriate to the situation of the patient can be considered morbid symptoms deserving of a high place in our search for the simillimum. Further, care should be taken not to prescribe on single symptoms (rubrics) however strong they may appear to be. Only when a Rubric matches with other marked symptoms of the patient can we be sure of its appropriateness in the case. In other words, we should prescribe on the basis of a *group of characteristic* symptoms which are components of the remedy selected.

We now give a set of typical general (not specific) questions which can induce the patient to reveal himself on those aspects of his personality on which we are focussing his attention, and are asking him to throw light on.

Group I Personality - Domineering; Go-getter and Group II Personality-Mild, Sensitive, Timid, Yielding	You must be quite ambitious to achieve whatever you have set your heart on. How do you react to obstacles in the way, natural or those created by others? What is the level of your anger when you are thwarted, or opposed? Will you go ahead with your plans and ideas in the teeth of opposition? What are your feelings towards such people who oppose? When confronted by a determined opponent, will you avoid confrontation and compromise as the better part of valour?
Group III Personality-Anxious, Fearful, Timid	Are there any circumstances which cause a high degree of anxiety in you? Are you troubled by fears of one type or another—of enemies, of robbers, of losing your job, of wife or husband being unfaithful, of incurable disease, of being alone, of misfortune, or loss of position in society, etc.?
-do-	
Group IV Personality-Restlessness	What type of activity gives you greatest pleasure?—Riding, rocking; dancing; travelling; Being carried (child); Quick, hurried work (slow people get on your nerves?).
Group V Personality-Planning, Thinking, Achievement	When are you in your happiest mood? What are the factors that add to or take away the pleasure of life? (planning; hard work—industriousness; company; jesting; occupation, diversion of mind; when you have taken revenge against the person who has offended you; when things are done to perfection - OR the OPPOSITE STATES).

Group VI Personality—Lascivious	Are you troubled by thoughts of sex? In what manner and how frequently?
Group VII Personality—Unsocial Behaviour	Are your inter-personal relationships with members of your family or associates in office or factory, or in society smooth or strained? To what extent, what you consider deficiencies on their part, disturb you mentally or influence your relationship or dealings with them? In what manner ?
Group VIII Personality—Unsocial traits Group IX Personality—Destructive	The signs and symptoms of Group VIII and Group IX Personalities have to be largely observed, or gathered from relatives or attendants of the patient.
Group X Personality—Sad, Melancholy	What is the effect on you of grief, shocks, disappointments and other adverse circumstances? (Brooding, Indifference, Anger, Averse to business, Despair, Weeping, Loathing at life, etc.?)
Group XI Personality-Unbearable shocks, effects of	Has there been any event in your life which has disturbed your mind very much? How have you reacted to them? How much are they affecting you today ?
Group XII Personality—Dullness	Have you any difficulty in understanding the matter you read or study; how is your clarity of thinking? Can you stand mental exertion? Any difficulty in remembering names, or what you have read, etc. ?

Unlocking the Patient's Mind

Group XIII
Personality—Imbeliles
Group XIV
Personality—Alienation

What is stated for Groups VIII and Group IX holds true of Groups XIII and XIV as well.

Group XV
Personality—Delusions

Do you have any fixed ideas, strong feelings or fears which your close relatives and well-wishers advise you to dismiss from your mind; telling you that they are unreal?

Group XVI
Personality—Habits; Obsessions

Do you have any compulsive habits like taking alcohol, drugs, tobacco smoking, or obsessive cleanliness resulting in constant washing of hands; or tormenting thoughts of various kinds?

Group XVII
Causations; Ailments From

Although appearing last in this Groupwise Classification, Ailments from various Causes, given from p 13 to 24 of Synthetic Rep. Vol.I must be invariably enquired into in every case.

Group XVIII
Aggr. and Ameliorations.

It is needless to say that unless the Aggravations and Ameliorations given under this Group (and others in the Report) are enquired into, the case cannot be said to be complete.

Questions on the above lines have the effect of jogging the patient's memory as well as jerking his feelings, and will *induce* him to *unburden* himself of his *hidden, suppressed* or *pent-up emotions*. It is our business then, to convert his situation into rubrics. A couple of cases are cited below illustrating how this is done. They will then be followed by the *narration* of patients' complaints or situations. The reader is required to convert them into appropriate rubrics, which are arranged serially and given in the second part of this section (section 8A).

Case I: A lady aged 35, who came for migraine since five years, was asked to tell everything about her life situation, and how she reacts to different situations. Her husband said that she feels hurt even from trifling remarks (*Offended easily; takes everything in bad part:* 791). How many persons are there in your family? She said they were in a joint family till a few years ago, but there was some serious disagreement with her sister-in-law and since then they are staying separately. The mother-in-law is staying with the SIL, who does not allow the MIL even to visit her, though they are not staying far. She was unhappy with this situation (*Discontented:* 403). She felt very much hurt by the MIL not coming to her house, and by her relatives commenting on it (*A.F. Honour, wounded:* 19). When questioned how she reacts to her anger in this situation, she said she beats her youngest daughter aged 7 years (*Strike, desire to:* 965). What else do you do when angry—shout, weep, sulk, or not talk? She said, except for beating my daughter for trifling reasons, I don't shout or weep. Yes, I suppress my anger (*A.F. Anger, suppressed:* 15), and do not talk (*Talk, indisposed to:* 987). I feel I have been discarded by my family (*Estranged from her family:* 444). I also tremble when angry (Kent's Rep.408). Her husband added, I know when she is angry; her face becomes red (*Face, discolouration red, anger after:* KR. 361). She was already opening up by now and added that she did not like the rudeness of her SIL (*A.F. Rudeness of others:* 22); she felt that her SIL was responsible for people treating her with scorn or contempt (*A.F. Scorn, being scorned:* 22). This lady turned out to be a *Staph—ysagria.* patient. A study of *Staph.* in Dr. M.L. Agarwal's "Materia Medica of the Human Mind" will bring to your notice many more outstanding, peculiar characteristics of this polychrest, which are worth committing to memory.

Case II: A lady came with the complaint that her elder sister, aged 56, a teacher had become very much depressed since about a year. She was not prepared to come out to meet the doctor or even to the market (*Going out, averse to:* 565) and would just sit down at home (*Sit inclined to:* 927), as if stupefied: (966). She was averse to company and was amel. when alone (146). Did not like to talk even with her husband (*Talk, indisposed to:* 986). When asked about the saddest event in her life, the sister said that the patient's only son, aged about 20, committed suicide by hanging, without leaving any clue as to his reason for doing so. Does she show or express her grief now, after 15 years of the event? She said 'no', but soon corrected herself saying that one day when she was taken to her friend's house about five years ago, she was asked how many children she had. She did not talk, but just lowered her head with sad face, suppressing her tears (*Grief, undemonstrative:* 569). Previously she was full of mirth, but now-a-days she was averse to jokes (*Jesting averse to:* 678). After studying these rubrics, it was found that *Cyclamen* was the lady's remedy. This remedy was confirmed by some further information. The patient found it difficult to concentrate on her teaching work (*Concentration difficult:* 155). Every night she was anxious as to how she will face the next morning's task of teaching in the school (*Work, aversion to mental:* 1096). She could not even do the cooking with the result that her husband had to help her in the kitchen. (*Indolence,* aversion to work, physical: 629).

Going through Dr. M.L.Agarwal's book, we found quite a number of rubrics which could represent her state of mind, which she would have expressed had she been communicative. For example: Anxiety of conscience, as if guilty of a crime: 69. Delusion, she has neglected her duty (to save her son from suicide): 327. Delusion, she has done wrong (Neglecting her son): 386. Forsaken feeling (by her son): 546.

Case III: The mother brought her 7 year old son with the complaint of catching cold easily. He was a fat boy who did not care about his appearance (*Obesity in children:* SR.II/394). (*Elegance, want of:* 437). How does he interact with other children in their building or at school? Oh, said the mother. He is horrible. Extremely obstinate, so much that he is unmanageable. (*Obstinate—chilly, refractory and clumsy:* 789). He is very sensitive when people, or children, laugh and joke among themselves, and he imagines that they thereby show a low opinion about him (*Offended easily*: 791). He is very attached to his father and a year ago, when his father had gone on a long business tour, he cried so much that the father had to be called back by wire (interpreted as *"Homesick"*: 576).

The following examples are not parts of cases, but are only given as exercises in interpretation. An earnest attempt to find the matching rubric will help the reader to think of these rubrics whenever a patient begins to unfold *similar* or *allied symptomatology.* The solutions are given at the end of this section, but should not be consulted before making a serious effort to identify the rubrics.

A few words of warning. These situations are only illustrative. There can be many other situations, (with the same essence, though) leading to the same rubric. Second, a particular situation could be interpreted into more than one rubric, *e.g.,* haughty, egotist, contradiction intolerant of. Third, For this reasons, we should not jump to any rubric unless we have made sure by asking "*Why* do you feel so" again and again, till he comes to the basic *reason* for his situation. For example, "*Why* can't you tolerate contradiction?" because it hurts my ego. Why are you so egoistic? My ego is satisfied only when I am praised. Is that sufficient? Certainly. So, basically he longs for the good opinion of others."

Complaint/Situation

1. Do you feel emotionally disturbed easily? When does it happen?
   I am very sensitive. I do not like to see accidents, murders or cruel scenes even on the T.V. Sometimes even tears come in my eyes on seeing or hearing sad occurrences.
2. Doctor, my brother has some serious mental breakdown from the time he has been suspended from his post as a police officer, on some false charges. He says he has committed a crime, and has to be restrained from running out of the house. He says he wants to hide somewhere.
3. What is your nature? Do you get along cordially with the people with whom you come in touch?
   Doctor, I will tell you everything, as I know that unless I tell you everything you cannot find the right remedy for me.
   I feel easily hurt; even if people just smile or make a harmless remark. I know I am wrong in feeling so, but it is my nature;
4. Then I go on thinking about it, wondering what those people may have been thinking about me.
5. Then again, if anyone is rough or rude or disrespectful to me, I can never forgive him, though I may have to meet him often on business.
6. I have a strong desire for sex; cannot avoid thinking of it all the time, though I have sex with my wife quite frequently.
7. You say that your son cannot concentrate on his studies. Is there any aspect of his temperament that you feel must be improved?
   Yes. Once he takes anything in his head it is very difficult to remove it. Now-a-days he is insisting on having a cycle. He is too young for it, and it is not essential. He gets very angry and does not accept any alternatives.
8. The husband said: You know my wife gets into bouts of depression. On such occasions, she will go on finding fault with me (not other people). Wife now said: I don't know why I do so. The fact is I do love him; he has been a great help to me in my depression. Any other husband would have sent away his wife.
   Another example: Why is it that my 7-year old daughter does quite the opposite things I ask her to do? I don't understand. If I ask her to read, she will go to play. If I tell her to go out and play, she sits down to read.
9. The patient was told: Many times things don't happen according to our wishes. How do you react to such situations? The husband of the patient promptly said, Oh, she goes to pieces if whatever she says, or wishes for, does not happen. Whatever she says I have to agree if there is to be peace in the house.

10. Patient said: Mr. A became very friendly with me and we decided to run a small business in partnership. But ever since we started the business, I find that all his promises and assurances are empty, in fact deceitful. He has cheated me. I realised it too late. I am easily taken in by people's words.
11. What is the rubric for Mr. A in the above example? Mr. A who has cheated the patient ?
12. I become very unhappy whenever thoughts of something bad happening come to my mind. For example, one day, early morning, as I opened my eyes, I felt that my father will die in a few days. I had no news then of his illness. The shocking event really happened......Again, one day when I was passing over the Mandovi bridge in Goa, I felt that the bridge will collapse in a few days. This also came to pass. This has happened many times.
13. My husband has been so kind and even charitable that he has given away money without even expecting its return. He has given Rs. 2 lakhs to his friend, and Rs.10,000 to a vegetable vendor, and so on. You will not believe that anyone can be so generous at one's own cost!
14. He thinks and behaves as if he is a moneyed man.
15. He is afraid that if he does not throw away his money in a show of generosity,- - -
16. - - he will lose his position in society - that people will have a low opinion about him
17. I plead with him to be careful with his money, but he does not care for the consequence of his action.
18. He insists on having his way, no matter what the consequences are.
19. Sorry to say this about my husband; he has no sense of right and wrong. He will even use violent means to support a wrong cause.
20. He does not hesitate to tell lies if he can thereby temporarily avoid an awkward situation, and to maintain what he thinks is his position in society.
21. Interaction between members of a family has very much to do with the health of each one of them. Please tell me what is the nature of your husband. Are you well adjusted?
    Patient says: We are married since 5 years. My husband becomes angry over small matters, but I keep my cool. What is the use of getting angry and quarreling?
22. I feel it is better to submit and keep quiet.
23. If there is a difference of opinion I think within myself whether I am in the right or in the wrong; may be wrong also!!

24. My son, this boy, is a terror to me, while he is like a meek sheep before his father. He dominate over me so much that I think it is better to yield to his wishes.
25. I am a doctor by profession, and I have to be pleasant and accommodating with my patients. I cannot afford to be hard with them. But at home, with my husband or children, I am firm and speak out when I am not satisfied.
26. I was very much attached to my father who died recently of sudden heart attack. She had tears in her eyes.
27. I am passing sleepless nights since then, for long hours.
28. I go on thinking why I was foolish not to listen to my father's advice about various matters. I don't know how to atone for my neglecting his wise counsel.
29. After being sleepless for quite some time, past midnight, my mind begins to thinks of what I must do to fulfil my father's dreams. I examine various alternative modes of action.
30. My mind becomes charged with many exalted ideas.
31. I get many ideas, my mind is full of ideas
32. My mind is active with many creative ideas.
33. A lady, 45, was very much harassed by her sister-in-law in the first few years of marriage. She bore it with great patience, but when it came to a bursting point they had sharp words, and SIL went away.
34. They have not been on talking terms since.
35. She was irritable by nature and was conscious of her position as the Landlady.
36. Some of her tenants were not well disposed towords her. One day, a tenants's son picked up a quarrel and called her a " prostitute". This made her furious.
37. She took this very much to heart, but did not allow her husband to talk to the offending family.
38. But she started behaving like an insane person—no food or drink, no sleep, but continuously prattling nonsensical words, occasionally
39. saying "rand" (prostitute)
40. What is your reaction when you feel insulted, or anyone does harm to your reputation or to your career?
    P.—If I get angry, I don't talk; I wait for the time when I get an opportunity, to take revenge.
41. What makes you really happy, and nurse that happy feeling for quite some time?

Unlocking the Patient's Mind 47

P. - Oh, My aim is to please everybody, and I am very happy when they praise me.
Example: An office-going lady said that, though tired after office work, she does everything at home to please her in-laws, but they treat her worse than a servant; call her "Shh.." instead of Smita. She is very happy in office; everybody appreciates and like her.

42. I am very particular to do my best in everything I do - in choice of words, expressions, speech. I am very concerned about my image.
43. Doctor, please help me. My son aged 8, is very backward. I teach him
44. a lesson ten times, but still he does not remember. He is very, very,
45. very slow. Even now, he can write words only alphabet by alphabet, e.g. "C-O-M-E", "S-W-I-M", "L-E-S-S-O-N". He trips on the feet of other children when playing, so they don't take him for their games. He has fallen many times.
46. I feel very much upset if anyone makes light of my remarks, or makes light-hearted jokes which I think are aimed at me.
47. I could not buy a costly saree (my wife's choice) on our wedding anniversary, and she acidly remarked I am a miser. Since then I have become bitter towards her,
48. My senior partner knows our business very well. Yet, as I am in the business for quite some time, I make some well thought out suggestions. If my partner opposes them, as he generally does, I feel extremely unhappy.
49. I feel, under these circumstances, like leaving the business; but as it is giving me good income, how can I leave it at this stage of my life. I am now nearly 50.
50. Has any event in your life left a lasting, bitter, angry feeling in you?
    I was holding a good position in our business, and my work was very much appreciated. Yet, people currying favour with the Chairman spoiled his mind against me and I was superceded by my juniors at
51. promotion time. I cannot forget the humiliation and frustration, unjustly inflicted on me. This injustice is rankling in my mind.
52. Tell me, young man, your mother is very depressed on your account. Can you tell me what is her expectation of you, and why you can't fulfil it.
    P.- I worked hard to get a Ph.D. in my thesis, but the publishers asked me to abridge it for printing. The work of abridgement has worn me
53. out so completely, that I can't muster up my will power to take up any work.
54. I have now a feeling that whatever I undertake will go wrong, and I will never succeed.

56. I have great fear of failure.
57. How is your sleep? I don't get sleep immediately I go to bed, as I used to do before marriage. Why? Because I go on thinking of the day's events; of all the remarks my MIL made showing her displeasure.
58. A lady, aged 35, started sobbing bitterly when she started telling her complaint to the doctor.
59. The doctor tried to pacify her, expressing sympathy and reassuring that whatever her problems, he will solve them with Homoeopathic medicine. She began to weep even more. Could not be consoled.
60. After some time (the doctor keeping silent), she regained her composure and said that she has a strong suspicion that her husband does not love her and he goes to other women.
62. The doctor asked, whether their sex life is normal.
    P.- How can it be normal? I get frightened at the very thought of relations.
63. Not only there is no pleasure in sexual act,
64. but there is great pain, which I cannot bear.
65. My child is very timid, gets frightened (starts) at any little noise
66. What was the state of your emotions during pregnancy.
    P:- I had great fear of death. It was my first pregnancy.
67. Mr. P: I have a peculiar vertigo which is worse lying and on closing eyes.
    Dr.: Yes, but tell me also why you have grown a beard? You were clean shaven only a few days ago.
    Mr.P- Well, I don't know why. I have a strange fear that I will injure myself if I shave.
68. Doctor, I pressed my husband hard to allow me to learn motor driving. I am now mid-way in the course and suddenly have developed some apprehension to continue the lessons. I have to be a safe driver, no !
69. Discontinuing the driving lessons will mean that I have wasted the amount, and I will have to find out means of recouping the loss.
70. I am feeling very anxious about my son, 7 year old. Instead of going out and playing with other children in the compound of our building, he just sits in a corner. He does not even play with toys given to him,
71. But my five year old daughter is quite the opposite. She observes and listens when elders are talking, and knows many things. She has an opinion on many things not normally seen at her age.
72. Ashwin (9 year old boy), how do you enjoy life with your school friends?
    I am not at all happy with the children; all of them are troublesome.

73. They want me to join them at play all the time, and if I don't agree they harass me in one way or another.
74. They use bad words and I feel very much troubled by them
75. The result is, I find myself prevented from doing my lessons well.
76. My 18 year old daughter had always topped the class, but in the last exam. she came third. Since then she has turned very religious - goes
77. to temple every day, prays before God, morning and evening.
78. A 20 year old boy came with the complaint that he has no self-confidence whatsoever. He is constantly scolded by his father and others at home in whatever he does. "I feel very much hurt by this treatment. I feel that I will not pass S.S.C. even after five attempts," he said.
79. Does your daughter have any special ability with which she impresses people?
    Yes, she has a great aptitude for imitating the voices of animals. She can also play the piano through her nose.
80. My brother behaves strangely when he is in the depths of depression. He tries to cut off his arm, and if any one tries to prevent him from
81. doing so, he bites them.
82. What do you do when you are very much depressed?
    You will not believe me Doctor; I don't get angry, nor do I cry. I plunge myself into my work, which helps me to overcome my depression.
83. My 8 year old son is having total loss of appetite and nausea. We have seen this happen every time when the examinations are approaching.
84. Sometimes he even gets fever.
85. How particular are you about neatness, order, system, etc? Oh, too much.
86. Neatness and tidiness are an obsession with me. I get furious if things are not in their place.
87. My mother is full of cares about her son and his children in America; and if she gets a letter from him, she will get anxious about her daughter in Calcutta. If they are all well, she will begin to feel anxious
88. about our neighbour's wife who has to cope with her job as well as her first pregnancy.
89. My five year old daughter is very obstinate. If her wishes are not fulfilled, she gets angry and begins throw out of the window whatever comes to hand.
90. But she is very bright in arithmetic, tables and calculations. If you ask her how much is 18 + 7, her answer (25) is immediate.

91. Her elder brother, now 9 year old, has no liking at all for even simple calculations. Special tuition has also failed to excite his interest in the subject. In fact, he hates maths.
92. What are your shopping habits, whether it is buying vegetables or sarees?

    Pt. looks at her husband and they both smile at each other. The wife says: I must always enquire about the price from two or three saree shops, or even vegetable vendors. My husband dislikes this, says I am wasting my time. He forgets that by doing so I am able to save a good amount.
93. My father met with a serious accident recently. His wounds are healed, but after coming from the hospital, he is behaving curiously, as if insane.
94. He recites Slokas (verses) of prayer;
95. says God is talking to him;
96. asks who we, his children, are
97. and becomes violent, trying to drive us all (our mother and we children) out of the house.
98. Does your child (2 year old) allow other children to join him when playing with his toys?

    Far from it. He does not allow other children even to touch his toys.
99. What is more, he takes the toys to pieces. They don't last even for a week. I don't know whether he takes pleasure in destroying them;
100. Or, it is due to his habit of tearing things, as he does with newspapers;
101. Or is it because he wants to know how the toys are made, what is inside them?
102. Whenever he knows that his friends are going to come, my son, 12 years old, hides his books, his birthday gifts. I don't know whether it is due to jealousy, or selfishness.
103. I entered politics with the object of serving people, to express peoples' hardships in the Parliament. I find that honesty does not pay. Some of my opponents are carrying all sort of false stories about me, to defame me.
104. My car has become a total wreck after being hit by an oncoming truck.
105. Thank God, I survived, but I feel the loss very much, which disturbs my sleep.
106. I get angry when so-called friends tell me not to brood over the loss.
107. A lady 40 years old said: I want to end my life. I am tired of my sufferings at the hands of my husband, an incorrigible drunkard.
108. My husband cannot pass a single hour without strong alcoholic drinks.

Unlocking the Patient's Mind

109. Under the influence of liquor he uses unmentionable bad words
110-111. He talks endlessly, going from one point to another.
112-112. He becomes extremely angry and begins to beat me
114. He beats me mercilessly, inhumanly. Doctor, I cannot stand this any more - see the wounds on my body.
115. She was weeping all this while, when telling about the sad story of life.
116. After seeing a couple making love freely in semi-darkness on the sea beach, I felt an irresistible urge to uncover my sister-in-law's blouse while she was in sleep (my brother, her husband being away on tour). I came to my senses in time, and withdrew from the shameful act. I was terrified at the thought that I may not be able to restrain myself from yielding to the temptation.
117. After this event, my conscience began to hurt me. I felt I was guilty of an unpardonable thought.
118. Ever since then I have a strong feeling of repentance.
119. The newspaper reports of my suspension on charges of corruption have hurt me deeply. I cannot have peace of mind till my innocence is proved in a Court. Till then how can I show my face to anyone?

    Another instance: I am afraid people will stare at me if I go out, and I tremble at the thought of being watched and talked about. This is my condition after appearance of the press reports that I was raped by college boys. Deep humiliation is my lot.
120. When the terrorists forced their way in the cashier's room in our Bank, both the cashiers faced them bravely, and being masters in Karate techniques, they overpowered the attackers.
121. A large number of guests landed in our house from Surat for my sister-in-law's marriage. Despite the over-crowding, my brother's family in the same town thought of living with us for full two days. No one dared to tell them to go back to their own house at least for the night. My wife however would not stand on ceremonies; at the risk of being considered immodest or insolent, she gently told them about our difficulties to accommodate them during night hours.
122. A lady came with her one year old child and complained that she is weeping all night and day since her father has gone to Europe on a business tour for a fortnight.
123. I hate to go on tours because the hotels are crowded and dirty; the service intolerable.
124. My daughter was full of joyful excitement and hilarity on the day of her engagement to a charming boy with bright future prospects.
125. She sang, even made her own verses.

126. She showed her tender affection for us, parents, for all that we have done for her and said she will never forget us even if she is far away from us with her husband.
127. My wife gave birth to a boy three days ago and since yesterday is talking incoherently. She does not allow me
128. to leave her; says that the police are after us, as she has committed a
129. crime. What has happened, for her to have these feelings?
130. She was very much attached to her mother, who was seriously ill at the same time that my wife was also advised total bed-rest due to some problems during pregnancy. In these circumstances, she could not be at the side of her mother in her last days. She feels she watched helplessly as her mother was dying.
131. She says again and again why God has chosen to punish her in this way? She is referring to her earlier miscarriage in the 8th month, and now the death of her mother.
132. A 7 year old boy was brought with the complaint of burning micturition. Two homoeopathic remedies had failed in the last six days. When asked about his nature, the mother said he was talkative all the time till he went to bed. She also said that she had admonished
133. him in the morning and to take "revenge", he struck her with his fist while sleeping at night.
134. The mother said, this is my 15 year old son studying in 10th Std. See, how thin he is; can't stand cold weather. They want children to learn public speaking, and he has to speak for ten minutes tomorrow. He is very nervous; says he will absent himself from school.
135. He is intelligent, but when will he learn to be more self-confident? So, your husband has had a stroke of left sided paralysis. Is he able to speak?
136. Yes, he does. But he tries our nerves. Whatever the cook does, he must find fault with the preparations, one way or another. He says the
137. cook killed her husband, and now she may do likewise to him also.
138. Do you have much pressure of work in the office? I do not consider it as pressure of work, though I work from 9 a.m. to 10 p.m. The fact is, though I am in charge of Finance, matters outside my portfolio such as Personnel, Legal, are referred to me.
139. But I don't feel the strain. I can work till late at night unmindful of delays in food. I enjoyed hard work.
140. Since his recent illness with typhoid, for which he was in bed for over a month, my son, aged 18 years, has become very dull;
141. He has become very slow in all his activities, bathing, eating;

142. If you ask him any questions, he takes quite some time to answer;
143. and when he answers, he does it very slowly.
144. My wife is carrying, now in the seventh month. We should be happy, but her behaviour is causing much anxiety. She cannot stand the slightest sounds, even of water flowing in the bathroom.
145. She says her parents are not dead, but are in England and after delivery she will go there to show her child to them, and they will introduce her to the Queen. No argument about the false ideas satisfies her.
146. and she begins to weep loudly.
147. She pleads with us to pray for her.
148. Mrs. P.S. You recently had a heart attack. Please tell frankly about all the stresses and shocks you have gone through. — Mine is a sad story.
149. I was very much attached to my only brother, and he died suddenly in an accident. And I was plunged in sorrow.
150. This made me indifferent to my household work.
151. Now I feel that I should not have neglected my work and put my husband and children to great inconvenience.
151(A). Because of my constantly talking and thinking about my brother and negligence of work, my husband became irritable. At this time I had a heart attack. I was kept in hospital, but I could see that my husband spared little time for me, and cared more for his business. I felt very much hurt.
152. Although the doctors say that my heart condition is stable, I have a terrible fear that I may die when I get another heart attack.
153. My daughter, married three years ago, returned to our house last week in a high state of nervous excitement.
154. She literally escaped form her husband's house, on over-hearing her mother-in-law's plans to beat her black and blue, as we could not meet her monetary demands.
155. She got terribly frightened, ran out of the house and took a taxi.
156. Since coming to our house she does not take interest in anything, even in music which she liked.
157. Yesterday she had a terrible headache, but she did not complain at all.
158. She is usually very sensitive to pains, but yesterday, we could not make out that she had a severe headache.
159. She is stunned and lying down as if her senses are blunted. It is difficult to awaken her for food.
160. does not even take food or drink.
161. My daughter, aged 40, does not go out of the house whatever the circumstances. I am 75 and yet I have to do marketing, etc. She says

"people will look at me and laugh, on seeing the hair loss on my forehead." It is really not so much; she thinks so. No argument helps. If I argue and ask how long she can can depend upon me to look after her, she weeps.

162. A lady, 73, had a heart attack, the pain in the heart preventing her from lying down. Being an active person taking part in various social activities even at this stage, she found it tiresome to be confined to bed. She started saying there is *no charm* in this type of life, and
163. began *praying* to God to take her away.
164. She desired, longed for death,
165. as she was tired of life.
166. When asked why she talked so much of death, which all family members do not want, she said she feels happy to face death.
167. Ever since my marriage my wife has been having one complaint or another. One day it is heaviness of her uterus, after some days it is her urination or pain in heart region, and if after treatment these complaints are relieved, she will be full of excitement,
168. with strong religious feelings (pooja, prayers, fasting, etc.), or alternately increased sexual desire even.
169. I am puzzled by these ever-changing wandering complaints.
170. When she has no physical complaints of uterus or heart, she is extremely hurried in everything as if she will be punished if she does not complete the work quickly.
171. She is so much hurried that she wants to do several things at the same time which, naturally, she cannot do.
172. One day I used the art of gentle persuation, and asked her to tell me without reserve or feelings of shame why she behaves in this erratic manner—hurry, religious or sexual excitement, etc. She told me that she thinks that sex is sinful and so she tried to spend time on religious activity. But in spite of herself she sometimes gets a violent sexual
173. desire with involuntary orgasm. At such time she must have natural sex to satisfy the instinct, or wear herself out through
174. hurried activity, occupation, etc.
175. Or I walk up and down fast to divert my mind from sexual excitement.
176. Sometimes I fear that these mental and physical troubles will make me
177. mad, as I afraid they are incurable.
178. A 37 year old lady came to Bombay from Punjab in a dazed condition. From the time she saw her brother-in-law being shot dead before.
179. her eyes, she would sit quietly
180. without talking to anyone,

Unlocking the Patient's Mind

181. as if buried in thought.
182. If she saw headlines of murders in the newspapers, she would say how long these cruelties will continue, and
183. weep for some time.
184. She was startled by any little noise; even some one knocking on the door, or the ringing of the door bell frightened her.
185. She began to avoid meeting people, saying that
186. they would observe her peculiar state of mind.
187. Yet, she had fear of being alone.
188. She asked repeatedly whether she will go mad.
189. A two year old girl was brought with the complaint of waking up, crying suddenly in sleep.
190. She screamed when the doctor looked at her, or tried to take her
191. pulse.
192. She would cry even if taken hold of and carried up and down.
193. She would stop weeping only if rocked in a cradle or a jhoola.
194. A 24 year old girl was in love with a young boy and they carried on their love affair for nearly a year. The girl began to slowly realize that the boy was having similar affair with other girls and
195. finally when she was able to catch him red—handed, broke off with him in a violent quarrel.
196. She could see no way of avenging this deception except to strongly wish for his death in an air crash, as he used to fly frequently to Dubai.
197. A 3 year old boy was suffering form mumps, and when the doctor entered the sick room, he began to cry loudly asking everyone in the room to go out.
198. He was very sensitive to pain; could not bear it.
199. So sensitive, he did not like to be asked about pain, or spoken to.
200. Inspite of the pain, he was asking repeatedly to be allowed to ride his tricycle, and wept loudly if advised not to ride when ill.
201. When at last the mother brought the tricycle in the room for him to ride, he rejected it.
202. He would even beat the mother on her face, when she tried to console him.

9

Rubrics

1. Horrible things, sad stories affect her profoundly (578). Cf. Cruelty in the cinema, children cannot bear to see. (190)
2. Delusion, criminal, he is a (260)
   Escape, attempts to, for fear of having committed a crime (441)
3. Offended easily, takes everything in bad part (791)
4. Brooding (115)
   Dwells on past disagreeable occurences (431)
5. Hatred of persons who had offended him. (571)
6. Lascivious (692)
   Thoughts sexual, day and night (1013)
7. Obstinate—resists the wishes of others. (790)
8. Contrary (perverse, self-willed) (185)
9. Contradiction, intolerant of (184)
10. Patient is: "CREDULOUS" (189); and "NAIVE" (782) Combine them.
11. DECEITFUL, sly (200) mislead with false pretentions. Cf. "CONTRADICTORY" to speech, intentions are. (185)
12. Clairvoyance (141)
13. Benevolence (109)
14. Delusion of wealth (382)
15. Squanders (949)
16. Despair, social position, of (396)
17. Heedless (573)
18. Dictatorial (398)
19. Moral feeling, want of (763)
20. Liar (706)
21. Mildness (743)
22. Yielding disposition (1102)
23. Introspection (649)
24. Contemptuous: hard for subordinates and agreeable, pleasant, to superiors or people he has to fear (182).
25. Same Rubric as for No. 24.
26. Grief (566)
27. Sleeplessness from grief (Sr.III/158)

28. Remorse (830)
29. Plans, making many (795)
30. Fancies, exhaltation of (466)
31. Ideas abundant, clearness of mind (594)
32. Activity, creative (9)
33. A.F. Anger suppressed (15)
34. Hatred of the persons who had offended him (571)
35. Haughty (572) Egotism (437)
36. A.F. honour wounded (19)
37. Egotism, self-esteem (437)
38. Insanity from mortification (642)
39. Loquacity insane (717)
40. Malicious, spiteful, vindictive (720)
41. Longing for the good opinion of others (712)
    Delusion, appreciated she is not (237)
42. Egotism, self-esteem (437) Cf. Conscientious about trifles (180)
43. Slowness (930)
44. Will- muscles refuse to obey the W. when attention is turned away (1095)
45. Fall, liability to (K1005)
46. Offended easily, takes everything in bad part (791)
47. Hatred, has bitter feelings for slight offences (571)
48. Contradiction, is intolerant of (184)
49. Helplessness, feeling of (574)
50. A.F. Mortification (21) Mortification, position loss of (21)
51. Injustice cannot support (633)
52. A.F. Work, mental (23)
53. Undertakes, lacks will power to undertake anything (1051)
54. Delusion, succeed, he cannot; does everything wrong (361)
55. Del., fail everything will (282)
56. Fear of failure. (499)
57. Brooding (115)
58. Weeping, telling of her sickness, when (1088)
59. Weeping, consolation agg. (1075) Inconsolable (607)
60. Suspicious, mistrustful (983)
61. Delusion, wife is faithless, and will run away from him (383)
62. Fear, at the thought of coition (in a woman) (484)
63. Coition enjoyment absent (SR. III/461)
64. Coition painful, from dryness of vagina. (SR.III/462)
65. Sensitivity to noise (901)

66. Fear of death, pregnancy during (491)
67. Fear, of cutting himself when shaving (486)
68. Anxiety, expected of him, when anything is (76)
69. Avarice (102)
70. Play, aversion to, in children; and sits in a corner (796)
71. Precocity (800)
72. Discontented (402)
73. Delusion, persecuted he is (335)
74. Rudeness, naughty children of (862)
75. Delusion, hindered at work he is (385)
76. Religious affections (827)
77. Praying (799)
78. Del. he is looked down upon (318) Del. he is dispised (265) Del. insulted he is (312)-fear of failure (490)
79. Imitation, mimicry; imitates voices and motions of animals (599)
80. Mutilates his body (780)
81. Bites everyone who disturbs him (112)
82. Occupation, diversion amel (790)
83. Fear before examination (498)
84. Anxiety, from anticipation of an engagement (64)
85. Fastidious (472)
86. Conscientious about trifles (180)
87. Cares, full of, about relatives (123)
88. Anxiety for others (86)
89. Anger, throws things away (38) Cf. Throws things away (1021)
90. Mathematics, apt (aptitude) for (728)
91. Mathematics, horror of (729)
92. Bargaining (107)
93. Insanity, religious (644)
94. Praying (799)
95. Delusion, God communication with, he is in (293)
96. Recognise, does not, his relatives (826)
97. Violent, chases family out of the house (1057)
98. Jealousy (674) Selfishness (895)
99. Destructiveness (397)
100. Tears things (996)
101. Inquisitive (633)
102. Jealousy (674)
103. Slander, disposition to (929)
104. Grief, losing objects after (568)

105. Brooding (115)
106. Consolation, kind words agg. (181) Anger, consoled when (32)
107. Suicidal, from despair about her miserable existence (976) Cf. Despair existence about, miserable (392)
108. Dipsomania (398)
109. Abusive (7)
110. Loquacity (713)
111. Speech, wandering (946)
112. Anger, violent (39)
113. Striking, desire to (965)
114. Brutality. drunkenness during (177)
115. Weeping, telling of her sickness, when (1088)
116. Fear, self-control of losing (522)
117 Anxiety of conscience, as if guilty of crime (69)
118. Remorse (830)
119. A.F. Shame (23)
120. Courageous (187)
121. Audacity (101)
122. Homesickness (576)
123. Disgust (411)
124. Ecstay (415)
125. Verses, makes (1055)
126. Sentimental (907)
127. Insanity, puerperal (644)
128. Delusion, pursued by the police (340)
129. Delusion Crime, committed he has (260)
130. Delusion, her brother fell overboard in her sight (250)
131. Delusion, God's vengeance, is the object of (294)
132. Loquacious (713)
133. Malicious, Spiteful, vindictive (720)
134. Timidity, appearing in public (1025)
135. Confidence, want of self (159)
136. Censorious, critical (126)
137. Suspicious, Mistrustful (983)
138. Boaster, braggart (115)
139. Or (if really a workaholic) Industrious, Mania for work (630)
140. Dullness, sluggishness, difficulty of thinking and comprehending, torpor (416)
141. Slowness (930)
142. Answers, reflects long (51)

143. Answers slowly (51)
144. Sensitive to noise of water splashing (905)
145. Fancies strange, pregnancy during (471)
146. Weeping aloud, sobbing (1070)
147. Praying, begged others to pray for him (800)
148. Sadness, despondency (864)
149 A.F.Grief (19)
150. Indifferent (609)
151. Delusion, neglected his duty, he has (327)
151(A). A. Delusion, neglected he is (327)
152. Fear of death, heart symptoms during (489)
153. Excitement, excitable (447)
154. Escape, attempts to (441)
155. A.F. Fright (18)
156. Indifferent to pleasures (620)
157. Indifference, complaint, does not (613)
158. Painlessness of complaints usually painful (SR. II/476)
159. Stupefaction, roused with difficulty (971)
160. Asks for nothing (101)
161. Hide, desire to, child thinks all visitors laugh at it and hides behind furniture (575)
162. Loathing at life (710)
163. Praying (799)
164. Death, desires (195)
165. Weary of life (1063)
166. Cheerful, death while thinking of (136)
167. Mental symptoms alternate with physical symptoms (742)
168. Religious affections alternating with sexual excitement (828)
169. Pains wandering (II/467)
170. Hurry, as by imperative duties (581)
171. Hurry, in occupations, desires to do several things at a time (582)
172. Religious (827)
173. Sexual desire violent with involuntary orgasm (III/608)
174. Must keep very busy to repress sexual desire (Phatak's M.M. 357)
175. Walks to and fro, cannot be amused by thinking or reading (582)
176. Fear disease, incurable of being (494)
177. Fear of insanity, losing his reason (506)
178. A.F. Fright (18) stupefaction, as if intoxicated (966)
179. Sit, inclined to (927)
180. Talk, indisposed to (986)

181. Absorbed, buried in thought (4)
182. Horrible things, sad stories, affect her profoundly (578)
183. Weeping, anxiety after (1073)
184. Starting from noise (956)
185. Company, averse to : avoids the sight of people (146)
186. Fear, confusion, that people would observe her (485)
187. Fear, alone, of being (477)
188. Fear, of insanity, losing his reason (506)
189. Shrieking during sleep (918)
190. Looked at, cannot bear to be (712)
191. Touched, averse to being (1028)
192. Weeping, child cries piteously if taken hold of or carried. (1073)
193. Rocking amel. (861)
194. A.F. Disappointed love (20)
195. Fear, betrayed being (482)
196. Jealousy, kill, driving to (675)
197. Irritable, sends the nurse out of the room (670)
198. Sensitive to pain (905)
199. Spoken to, averse to being (948)
200. Obstinate (787)
201. Capriciousness (120)
202. Striking, in children (964)

10
Repertory Page-wise Rubrics with the corresponding Serial number of the Complaint/Situation given in Section 8

Page No. of Repertory	Rubric	Complaint No. in Sec. 8
4	Absorbed, buried in thought	181
7	Abusive	109
9	Activity creative	32
15	A.F. Anger, suppressed	33
18	A.F. Fright	155-178
19	A.F. Grief	149
19	A.F. Honour, wounded	36
20	A.F. Disappointed love	194
20	A.F. Jealousy	194
21	A.F. Mortification	50
21	Mortification, from loss of position	50
23	A.F. Work, mental	52
23	A.F. Shame	119
32	Anger consoled when	106
38	Anger, throws away things	89
39	Anger, violent	112
51	Answers, reflects long to	142
64	Anxiety from anticipation of an engagement	84
51	Answers slowly	143
69	Anxiety of conscience, as if guilty of a crime	117
76	Anxiety, expected of him, when anything is	68
86	Anxiety for others	88
101	Audacity	121
101	Asks for nothing	160
102	Avarice	69
107	Bargaining	92
109	Benevolence	13
112	Bites everyone who disturbs him	81
115	Brooding	5-57-105
115	Boaster, braggart	138

117	Brutality, drunkenness during	114
120	Capriciousness	201
123	Cares full of, about relatives	87
126	Censorious, critical	136
136	Cheerful, death, while thinking of	166
141	Clairvoyance	12
146	Company, averse to, avoids the sight of people	185
159	Self-Confidence, want of	135
177	Brutality, drunkenness during	114
180	Conscientious about trifles	42-86
181	Consolation, kind words agg.	106
182	Contemptuous—hard for subordinates and agreeable, pleasant to superiors or people he has to fear	24-25
184	Contradiction intolerant of	9-48
185	Contradictory to speech, actions are	11
185	Contrary	8
187	Courageous	120
189	Credulous	10
190	Cruelty in the cinema, children cannot bear to see	1
195	Death, desires	164
200	Deceitful	11
237	Del. she is not appreciated	41
250	Delusion, brother fell overboard in her sight	130
260	Del. he is a criminal	2
260	Del. crime he has committed	129
265	Del. he is despised	78
282	Del. everything will fail	55
293	Del. God, he is in communication with	95
294	Del. of wealth	14
294	Del. God, is object of God's vengeance	131
312	Del. insulted, he is	78
315	Brooding	57
318	Del. he is looked down upon	78
327	Del. neglected his duty, he has	151
327	Del, he is neglected	151-A
340	Del. pursues by the police, he is	128
335	Delusion, persecuted he is	73
361	Del. succeed he cannot	54
382	Del. of wealth	14
383	Del. wife is faithless	61
385	Del. hindered at work, he is	75
392	Despair about her miserable existence	107
396	Despair, social position of	16
397	Destructiveness	99

398	Dictatorial	18
398	Dipsomania	108
402	Discontented	72
411	Disgust	123
415	Ecstasy	124
416	Dullness, Sluggishness	140
431	Dwells on past disagreeable occurrences	4
437	Egotism, self esteem	35-37-42
441	Escape, attempts to	2-154
447	Excitement, Exciteable	153
466	Fancies, exhaltation of	30
471	Fancies, strange, during pregnancy	145
472	Fastidious	85
477	Fear, being alone of	187
482	Fear, being betrayed	195
484	Fear at the thought of coition (in woman)	62
486	Fear, cutting himself when shaving	67
489	Fear of death, heart symptoms during	152
490	Fear of failure	78
491	Fear of death, pregnancy during	66
498	Fear before examination	83
485	Fear, confusion, that people will observe her	186
490	Fear of failure	78
494	Fear, disease, incurable of being	176
499	Fear of failure	56
506	Fear of insanity	177-188
522	Fear, self-control, of losing	116
566	Grief	26
568	Grief, losing objects after	104
571	Hatred of persons who offended him	6-34
571	Hatred, has bitter feelings for slight offences	47
571	Hatred, unmoved by apologies	45
572	Haughty	35
573	Heedless	17
574	Helplessness	49
576	Home-sickness	122
575	Hide, desire to, child thinks visitors laugh at it, and hides behind furniture	161
578	Horrible, sad stories affect him profoundly	1-182
581	Hurry, as by imperative duties	170
582	Hurry in occupation, desire to do several things at a time	171
594	Ideas abundant	31
582	Walks to and fro, cannot be amused by thinking or reading	175
599	Imitation, mimicry	70

600	Precocity	68
607	Inconsolable	59
609	Indifferent	150
613	Indifferent, does not complain	157
620	Indifferent to pleasures	156
630	Industrious, mania for work	139
633	Injustice, cannot support	51
633	Inquisitive	101
642	Insanity, from mortification	38
644	Insanity, religious	93
644	Insanity, puerperal	127
649	Introspection	23
670	Irritable, sends the nurse out of the room	197
674	Jealousy	98-102
675	Jealousy, kill driving to	196
675	Jealousy, between children	95
692	Lascivious	5
620	Indifferent, to pleasures	156
706	Liar	20
710	Loathing at life	162
712	Longing for the good opinion of others	41
712	Looked at, cannot bear to be	190
717	Loquacity, insane	39
713	Loquacity	110-132
720	Malicious	40-133
728	Mathematics, aptitude	90
729	Mathematics, horror of	91
742	Mental symptoms alternate with physical	167
743	Mildness	21
763	Moral feeling, want of	19
780	Mutilates his body	80
782	Naive	10
787	Obstinate	200
790	Obstinate, resists the wishes of others	7
791	Offended easily, takes everything in bad part	3-46
790	Occupation amel.	82
795	Plans, making many	29
796	Play, aversion to, in children	70
799	Praying	77-94-163
800	Praying, begged others to pray for him	147
800	Precocity	71
826	Rocognise, does not, his relatives	96
827	Religious affections	76-172
827	Refuses to take the medicene	94

Repertory Page-wise

828	Religious affection alternating with sexual excitement	168
830	Remorse	118-128
861	Rocking amel.	193
862	Rudeness, haughty children, of	74
864	Sadness, despondency	148
895	Selfishness	102
901	Sensitive to noise	65
905	Sensitive to pain	198
905	Sensitive to noise of water splashing	144
907	Sentimental	126
918	Shreiking, during sleep	189
929	Slander, disposition to	103
927	Sit inclined to	179
930	Slowness	43-141
946	Speech wandering	111
948	Spoken to, averse to being	199
949	Squanders	15
956	Starting from noise	65-184
964	Striking, in children	202
965	Striking, desire to	44-113
966	Stupefaction	178
971	Stupefaction, roused with difficulty	159
976	Suicidal, despair from	107
983	Suspicious	60-137
986	Talk, indisposition to	180
946	Speech, wandering	111
927	Sit, inclined to	179
996	Tears things	100
1013	Thoughts, sexual, day and night	5
1021	Throws things away	89
1025	Timiditdy, appearing in public	134
1028	Touched, averse to being	191
1051	Undertake, lack of willpower to undertake anything	53
1055	Verses, making	125
1057	Violent, chases family out of the house	97
1063	Weary of life	165
1068	Weeping, telling of her sickness, when	58
1075	Weeping, consolation agg.	59
1070	Weeping aloud, sobbing	146
1073	Weeping, anxiety after	183
1073	Weeping, child cries piteously if taken hold of or carried	192
1088	Weeping, when telling of her sickness	58-115
1095	Will, nuscles refuse to obey the will when attention is turned away	44
1102	Yielding, disposition to	22

Rubrics from Other repertories

Syn. R.II/476	Painlessness of complaints usually painful	158
II/476	Pains, wandering	169
III/402	Coition, painful from dryness of vagina	64
III/461	Coition, enjoyment absent (Female)	63
III/608	Sexual desire violent, with involuntary orgasm	173
Kent's Rep. 1005	Fall, liability to	45
Phatak's M.M. - 357	Must keep busy to repress her sexual desire	174

11

Do Not Neglect Objective Symptoms

What is the relevance of objective symptoms in the *totality*? The answer will be found when we understand the true meaning of totality. Dr. Guy Beckley Stearns, quoting Joseph T. O'connor, described it as the unity of the life-energy in a body. It is the same life, he said, whether it expresses itself in the nervous, digestive, muscular, or any other system. There is no separate life for the different organs or parts. Each part must express the nature of the whole. Nearly every one would recognise an oak tree and most of us would recognise oak wood in furniture, an oak leaf, an acorn, or the bark of the oak tree. All of these parts partake of the nature of the oak. So, in each case of illness, each symptom partakes of the nature of the remedy that corresponds to the whole case. After advising that the most characteristic symptoms in each part and function of the body should be taken together, Dr. G.B. Stearns observed: The most valuable symptoms are those which are objective. These guide the experienced man to some of his most brilliant prescriptions. A valuable object lesson to students is to lead them to prescribe for a case without asking a question. The students in a hospital began the experiment of observing a patient. They observed that he was rather a grouch and didn't like to talk; he was stubborn and irritable, and was easily offended. Repertorial study of these mental characteristics and a reference to the Materia Medica led to Sulphur which benefited him.

Dr. C.M. Boger considered an article "Objective Symptoms" worthy enough for translation into English. In this the author, Dr. Halle has written at length on the importance of Objective symptoms. Readers may read it on page 21 of Jan-Feb. 1982 Issue of *Homoeopathic Heritage*. In this article the author says, "Every illness which we or the laity may observe with our five senses, conclusively depicts an objective symptom. Among those are found exactly those which are of decisive import in the choice of the remedy." He then cites a case of pneumonia in which, put briefly, three objective symptoms were Agg. observed, viz. Agg. from lying on the side (can only lie on the back); from warm wrapping (he repeatedly put his arms out of the covers), as well as amelioration when lying with the head high (with two pillows). These did not arise in the imagination of the patient, and objectively individualise our case of pneumonia. The remedy chosen cured the case.

The author goes on to say, "objective manifestations of the greatest importance appear in sub-acute and chronic as well as acute sickness. It is in these particularly that homoeopathy, when rightly handled, glories in her triumph. If we rightly observe and learn to use these symptoms, we will enjoy the greatest satisfaction in treating chronic cases. Light and simplicity at once come into the chaos of the most inexplicable and unheard of complaints with the consequence that we can, without reserve, place our reliance on such symptoms..."

"He who glances through the Materia Medica will find that almost every remedy possesses a number of typical objective symptoms which do not repeat the same combination under any other... But he who, from this, believes that he can neglect real subjective symptoms (even if they seem unsafe and not indicative) will find it a costly mistake for they belong to the disease picture just as the objective ones... Both have the same weight. We need all the evidences, in every case, in order to heal quickly, safely and pleasantly."

We shall now present a few **objective symptoms** which we could gather at short notice.

1. A child with its open mouth, with a stupid expression, and to avoid our gaze, it shrinks behind its mother from whence it timidly observes us?
   -Baryta carb.
2. An obese lady slowly ascends the steps laboriously, gasping for breath, while she wipes beads of sweat from her forehead and face.
   -Calc. carb.
3. A thin, lean man with poorly; washed clothes, drooping shoulders red eyelids, seeks a seat under the fan.   -Sulphur.
4. Gestures, picks at bed clothes   SR.I/558
5. Gesticulates while talking   SR.I/565
6. Each time a patient comes you find him dressed in gaudy, colourful clothes; each time different. You begin to wonder at his "Tastelessness in dressing"   SR.I/995
7. Indifference to personal appearance   SR.I/620: SULPH.
8. Indifference to remain naked :   619: HYOS.
9. Tastelessness in dressing: 995: (II remedies)
10. Talks- does not care whether anyone listens: 995: Sticta.
11. Tears her hair: 996: Bell, Lil-t, Tarent.
12. Speech: (abrupt; childish; foolish; hasty, etc.): 924-946.
13. Throws things away: 1021.
14. Weeping in sleep   1086
15. Late, always too   694 - Calc., Plat., Puls., Sil.

Do not neglect

16. Begging, entreating: 109
17. Bite, desire to 110 - BELL., STRAM, etc.
18. Moonlight, mental symptoms from: 763
19. Rocking agg. or amel. 861
20. Washing, mania for cleanness 1062
21. Irony, satire, desire for 650
22. **Face:** Expression: Anxious; besotted, frightened; old looking; sickly; suffering: KR. 374-375
    Wrinkled forehead : KR. 396.
    Greasy, face: KR. 375
    Discoloration: Bluish; dark; dirty looking; pale: circumscribed; glowing red; one side pale, the other red; red, with toothache; Lips red; yellow (jaundice): KR.357-364.
23. **Tongue:** Flabby (KR.405); Mapped (407)
24. **Mouth:** Odour offensive (409); Open, sleep during (409)
25. **Tongue:** Cracked, fissured: KR. 399
26. **Gums:** Detached from teeth: (KR.399)
27. **Tongue:** Coated (discoloration): black blue, brown; red; white; glistening; yellow., yellow base. KR.400-403.
28. **Teeth:** Caries, decayed, hollow: KR.431
    discolored black: KR.431
29. **Throat:** Membrane, exudation, diphtheria: KR.455
    Elongated uvula: KR.451. Enlargement of Tonsils (451)
    Inflammation, tonsils: 454
30. **Vomiting:** Bile, blood, coffee grounds like; everything; fecal; food; frothy, liquids; milk; mucus; sour; stringy, water; worms; yellow. (535-540)
31. **Abdomen:** Dropsy (546). Enlarged liver; mesenterics; spleen. (546). hard (550). hernia (552) Retraction of abdomen (600).
    Nose: Boring in, with fingers (324). Pricking nose; until it bleeds; in brain affections (348).
    Nostrils, dilated during experation: Ferr. (329)
    Discharges: bloody; copious; crusts, scabs inside; greenish; offensive, purulent, suppressed; thick, viscid; watery, yellowish green; posterior nares (329-334)
    Fan like motion of alae nasi (of wings); in pneumonia; (340)
32. **Stool:** Hard or soft. Copious or Scanty. Knotty and Sheepdung like. Colour: light-coloured, or brown, or bloody, or cream-coloured, dark or green; white or yellow; forcible or shooting out; Mocuous. (635-644).

33. **Urine:** Albuminous; Alkaline; bloody; Casts, epithelial, fat drops. Cloudy. Colour: brown, dark, greenish, pale; blood-red; dark-red. Smoke-colour, chalky, dark yellow. Copious or Scanty. Sediment cloudy, flocculent; gelatinous; mucous; sand, gravel. Milky urine. (680-692)

34. **Genitalia:** Atrophy of penis or testes (693). Hydrocele (699). Inflammation: spermatic cord (699). Retraction penis; testes (709). Swelling: spermatic cord (712).

    Female: ovaries, dropsy, enlarged, swollen (717).

    Leucorrhoea: albuminous, greenish, milky, purulent, ropy or stringy, tenacious, thick, transparent, white or yellow (720-723). Rigidity of os during labour (744).

35. **Larynx And Trachea:** Voice: barking; hollow; husky; lost; toneless, tremulous, weak, whispering. Whistling (758-761).

36. **Respiration:** Accelerated. Abdominal. Arrested; Asphyxia. Asthmatic. Deep, desire to breathe. Difficult. Irregular (774). Loud (774). Panting. Rattling (774). Sighing; snoring; sterterous, stridulous, wheezing, whistling (776).

37. **Cough:** Asthmatic, Constant. (784). Croupy; Deep-sounding (785). Hacking; hoarse, hollow (793). Loose. Paroxysmal. Suffocative.(806). Cough agg. by talking (807). Tormenting, violent. (809). Whooping (810).

38. **Expectoration:** Colour: Bloody, brownish, Grayish, Greenish (812-821) Rusty, Transparent, white, yellow. Milky.

    Consistency: Frothy, gelatinous, granular, lumpy, mucous, purulent, stringy, thick, tough, viscid, watery.

    Taste: Bitter, greasy, nauseous, putrid, salty, sour, sweetish.

    Copious or Scanty.

    Difficult (Hard); or Easy (Hawked up).

39. **Chest:** Cracks of nipples (828). Indurations & Nodules of mammae (835; 838).

40. **Extremities:** Emaciation or diseased limb (985)

    Excoriation, bends of joints, etc. (1004). Gangrene (1009). hang down, Letting limbs; agg. or amel. (1009). Perspiration of palm (1182); of foot (1183); of sole (1184). Restlessness of feet (1188). Trembling of hands on holding objects (1212); when carrying something to the mouth (1212).

41. **Sleep:** Position during sleep: On Abdomen (SR.III-54-55); Arms on abdomen; on back; hands crossed over abdomen (PULS); Head low, with (Dig. Nux-V;) Head low, impossible (III-58). Changed frequently,

genupectoral (III 59). hard, every position seems (Laur., mag-c.,phos). On the knees, with face forced into the pillow (III-62). On left side; on right side. (65).

42. **Pulse:** Abnormal; accelerated (1393). Faster than the heart beat (KR. 1394). Full. hard. Imperceptible (1395). Irregular. Slow. Small. Soft. Tremulous. Weak (KR.1396-7).

43. **Eyes:** pupils contracted or dilated (KR. 263). Protrusion of eyes. Eyes staring. Redness. Sunken. Movements, convulsive, etc. (246); turned up or down (266). yellowness (jaundice)

44. **Miscellaneous:** Dr. Sarabhai Kapadia reported a case of heart attack helped by Aurum, after observing that the patient was answering in questions, to whatever questions he was asked. (SR.I-51. and Kent's Rep. 70: Questions, speaks continuously in).

45. Patient starts talking to the doctor abruptly. Does not even wait for the doctor to raise his head and look at him to listen: patient is very anxious and impatient.

46. Patient looks back over his shoulders repeatedly while telling his case to the doctor= He has something to hide; Anxiety of conscience, as if guilty of a crime.

47. While narrating his complaints, patient suddenly rises and walks about; says, sorry, I am restless while sitting= Restless, sitting while (SR.I-856).

48. Patient complains of severe abdominal pain—kneels on the ground and presses his abdomen hard on the edge of the cot for relief. = Stannum.

49. Boy is playing about as if nothing had happened, though the parents complain that he has been having diarrhoeaic stools 4-5 times a day. = Diarrhoea, weakness, without (KR.615)- Phos. ac.

50. Child does not allow you to feel his pulse, or examine his chest with stethoscope = Touch, averse to.

51. A case of bronchitis with loose rattling cough, and inability to raise the expectoration was very much helped, bringing out profuse expectoration, on observing that he had flapping of alae nasi with agg. of cough, etc. when lying on back; he must sit up to breathe or cough=Antim. tart.

52. Jaundice with slow, weak pulse was described by Dr. Sarabhai Kapadia as the briefest totality of Digitalis.

53. Patients forgets words while speaking = Thoughts vanish.

54. Child does not allow mother to be away from her at any time; mother cannot even go to the toilet = Clinging to persons of furniture. Child

always hold the hand of the mother: (Clinging)== Bismuth.
55. Patient dirty; face greasy and enjoys sitting in the sun = Psor.
56. Patient replies all questions with one word (yes, or no) = Speech, monosyllabic (942).
57. Patient turns face away form light during fever == photophobia.
58. Patient very well dressed, with neat pressed, spotless clothes == Fastidious.
59. While coughing, patient brings knees and chest together == Cough violent - spasmodic perking of head forward and knees upward (KR.810) == Theridion
60. Child wants to be carried; will be quiet only when carried ==? Carried fast, or slowly. (KR.10).
61. Complaints agg. by slightest motion, amel. by absolute rest and lying on the painful side == Bryonia.
62. Body surface cold to touch, yet cannot bear to be covered. Throws off coverings == Camph (Med. Sec.)
63. Cyanosis; cold extremities, cold breath, cold sweat. Vital force exhausted. Desires to be constantly fanned. == Carb. Veg.
64. Extreme paleness; red parts become white == Ferr.
65. All orifices of body very red; anus red, excoriated = Sulph.
66. Distinct blue line along margin of gums. Excessive and rapid emaciation = Plumbum
67. Cold sweat on forehead; profound prostration = Verat. alb.
68. Ulcers punched out, deep, perforating, round—Kali bich.
69. Pulse slow in recumbent posture, quick on motion, irregular and dicrotic on sitting up == Digitalis.
70. Child worse (afraid) when rocking or being dangled up and down = Borax.
71, Loquacity during fever; chilly, wants cover in all stages of fever.
72. Gall- Stones colic, amel. by rubbing over liver region =Podo.
73. Cross, snappish; averse to being spoken to or touched; cannot bear anyone near him. = Cham.
74. Cross, fretful; cries if looked at or touched; dread of bathing = Antim. curd.
75. Eruptions with thick crusts, with pus beneath. Intolerable itching changes place on scratching = Mezerium.
76. Cough - Hands, must hold chest with both, while Coughing
Cough - Holding pit of stomach amel.
Cough - holding abdomen Amel.   KR. 792.

Do not neglect

77. Chewing motion of jaw before attack of opilepsy =Calc. c.(KR.356)
78. Head, jerks the head clear of the pillow while lying = STRAM.
79. Sour smell of whole body, even after washing or bathing = RHEUM
80. Pulse abnormally rapid, out of all proportion to temperature = PYROGEN
81. Stool large, hard, lacerating anus; painful, extracts cries =Lac.def.
82. Red sand in urine = Lycopodium
83. Stool, knotty hard, crumbles at the verge of anus = Mag.mur.
84. Baglike swelling between upper eyelids and eye - brows =Kali c.
85. Pricking at the nose or lips until they bleed = Arum trip. Screams with pain, yet keeps up the boring.
86. Heat of upper part of body, coldness of the lower part = Arn.
87. Sudden noise (Crackers, door - bell) frightens = Borax.
88. Face cold, blue, pale, covered with cold sweat = Ant. tart.
89. Cough violent paroxysms follow each other rapidly. Scarcely able to get breath = Dros.
90. Appetite ravenous, with emaciation or marasmus =KR. 479
91. Nails thorny, deformed, thickened, crippled =KR. 978.
92. Heart - holds hand over heart during violent pain extending to scapula and neck == Naja.
93. Excoriation, bends of joints == KR.1004.
94. Clenching thumbs in epilepsy == KR.956.
95. Awkwardness, hands,drops things =KR.953.
96. Coldness, hand, one hot other cold = KR.959.
97. Coldness, feet, icy cold = KR.963
98. Contraction, thigh, hamstrings = KR.967.
99. Twitching, eyelids =KR.269
100. Lockjaw (trismus) = KR. 394
102. Skin, discoloration yellow, jaundice = KR.1307.

Appendix A
Excerpts from The Trend of Thought Necessary for the Comprehension and Retention of Homoeopathy
(Kent's Minor Writing: P. 598)

I desire to have my friends shun some things leading away from Hahnemann's thoughts... The tendency to depart from his methods is the largest danger of pupils today... The idea of going from centre to circumference always, from first to last, from things prior to things ultimate. I have thought along this line for twenty-five years, and must make it most forcible in maintaining the idea of homoeopathy.

First, the centre of man is his loves... his Cravings... Proceeding toward the circumference, work out those remedies related to the disordered affections first. Any remedy not in this group cannot cure. The second point for study is the intellectual functions, the reasoning faculties... Consult the most important, those most strange first.

Next in importance are the physical generals—they cannot be cured with remedies that do not have the mental conditions; the patient's relation to heat and cold... What has this to do with the hip joint, the kidneys, the liver...? Nothing, yet, these things relate to the man as a unit, his bodily condition in its entirety. They are generals... Many remedies have the modalites of the part differing from those of the patient. Take first things first; the patient first before his parts.

Perhaps only one remedy in the list of mental symptoms is worse from heat (physical general). Then why need you care about the particulars. You have the man himself, and the particulars will take care of themselves. Most cases of hip-joint disorder cured by me in the past twenty-five years were cured by remedies not in the hip-joint list. Those in the list may not cure another hip-joint case.

A man with rectal ulcer, who was advised operation, consulted me. A persistent mental symptom in him was the need for intense restraint to prevent himself from self-destruction. Natrum Sulph. has this symptom, but has no rectal ulcer recorded. A few other symptoms together with this strong mental, led to the use of Nat. Sulph. and he had no more hemorrhages. *Find the remedy for the patient and it will cure him, and the particulars will disappear though none of them were in that remedy...* Although a remedy may not be known to fit the pathology, if it fits the patient, that remedy will cure the patient. By becoming expert in this method you can do wonderful things.

By the Boenninghausen and Boger method, there is no opportunity to distinguish between the patient and the particulars. This method has obscured Hahnemann's homoeopathy: the patient first, focusing on things strange, rare and peculiar. These do not relate to the particulars (the parts affected). Guided by the symptoms of the patient you can cure inflammation of any part even if that remedy has not produced inflammation of that sort.

References

Oraganon of Medicine: Samuel Hahnemann. B. Jain Publishers P. Ltd. New Delhi.

The Genius of Homoeopathy: Stuart Close. B. Jain Publishers.

Lectures on Homoeopathic Philosophy: J.T. Kent B. Jain Publishers.

The Prinçiples and Art of Cure by Homoeopathy: H.A. Roberts. B. Jain Publishers.

Use of the Repertory and How to use the Repertory: J.T. Kent. B.Jain

On the Comparative Value of Symptoms in the Selection of the Remedy: Robert Gibson Miller. B.Jain

Repertorising: Margaret Tyler and Dr. John Wier, B. Jain Publisher

Totality of Symptoms: A Pulford. Indian Journal of Homoeopathic Medicine ( ), N. Gadkari Marg, Vile Parle (W), Bombay, 56.

Kent's Minor Writings on Homoeopathy (P. 142: What is Homoepathy; Page 477: Representative Symptoms).

Recommended Essental Reading

Besides the above "References", the reader is strongly advised to study the following articles in Kent's Minor Writings as eessential reading:

P. 438 - The Administration of the Remedy.

P. 474 - Observations regarding the selection of the potency.

P. 640 - Use of Potencies. Application of Remedies to sickness.

P. 628. - Successful Prescribing -The Essential.

Probing The Mind And Other Guiding Symptoms
A Blueprint for Success

"Probing the Mind and other Guiding Symptoms" by Shri. S.M.Gunavante makes interesting and useful reading. It is true, searching for mental symptoms or mental state, is a very difficult task for novices as well as seasoned practitioners. It needs a deep study of the complex human mind and personality. The Group-wise classification of personalities in Section 7 greatly reduces the task of the physician and gives him, helping hand in arriving at, reasonably correct disposition of mind. I must say that Shri Gunavante has done a very valuable scanning of the existing literature to present the relevant data in the right place for the benefit of practitioners. He has done well to include details of other 'Guiding symptoms' also, thus making this a complete case- taking guide. This booklet is a must for everyone who wishes to practise homoeopathy rationally and successfully.

—*Dr. K.P.Muzumdar,*
Hon. Prof.C.M.P.Homoeopathic
Medical College,Bombay.Former Director,
National Institute of Homoeopathy,G O I, Calcutta.

About the Author

I have admired Mr. Gunavante's dedication for the spread of Homoeopahty, for nearly a decade. Be it a seminar, a meeting, a case study or a journal, he is in the forefront, and yet a silent worker. A popular teacher of Homoeopathy, he has been actively associated with the starting and running of the Homoeopathic teaching and training classes under Dr. Subodh Mehta Medical Centre, Khar, since 1981, under Dr. V.R.Shah Medical Centre Marine Drive, since 1985 and under R & K T.Thakur Trust in Chembur since 1988. He is an active member of the Homoeopathic Convention Committee which has organised one seminar a year since 1985. About his book, "Introduction to Homeopathic Prescribing" (a text book for the Classes organised by our centre) Dr. Karl Robinson, Editor, Journal of the American Institute of Homoeopathy says: "It appears to include virtually all points of view on all areas of Homoeopathy. I doubt anyone has done so thorough and good as job if it." Now "Probing the Mind...." I am sure will help practitioners to attain higher levels of efficiency than ever with its refrehsingly practical guidance -with over example for interpreting symptoms into Rubrics.

—*Dr.S.K.Mankad, LCEH,CHA (Bom)*
Medical Executive & Chief Homoeopathic Physician,
Dr. Subodh Mehta Medical Centre. 16th Road, Khar,
Bombay